Heart Failure and Transcatheter Aortic Valve Replacement

Editor

NICOLE JUDICE JONES

CRITICAL CARE NURSING CLINICS OF NORTH AMERICA

www.ccnursing.theclinics.com

Consulting Editor
DEBORAH GARBEE

June 2022 • Volume 34 • Number 2

ELSEVIER

1600 John F. Kennedy Boulevard • Suite 1800 • Philadelphia, Pennsylvania, 19103-2899

http://www.theclinics.com

CRITICAL CARE NURSING CLINICS OF NORTH AMERICA Volume 34, Number 2
June 2022 ISSN 0899-5885, ISBN-13: 978-0-323-98759-2

Editor: Kerry Holland
Developmental Editor: Ann Gielou M. Posedio

Critical Care Nursing Clinics of North America (ISSN 0899-5885) is published quarterly by Elsevier Inc., 360 Park Avenue South, New York, NY 10010-1710. Months of issue are March, June, September, and December. Business and Editorial Offices: 1600 John F. Kennedy Blvd., Suite 1800, Philadelphia, PA 19103-2899. Periodicals postage paid at New York, NY and additional mailing offices. Subscription prices are $160.00 per year for US individuals, $593.00 per year for US institutions, $100.00 per year for US students and residents, $206.00 per year for Canadian individuals, $611.00 per year for Canadian institutions, $230.00 per year for international individuals, $611.00 per year for international institutions, $115.00 per year for international students/residents and $100.00 per year for Canadian students/residents. To receive student/resident rate, orders must be accompanied by name of affiliated institution, data of term, and the *signature* of program/residency coordinator on institution letterhead. Orders will be billed at individual rate until proof of status is received. Foreign air speed delivery is included in all *Clinics* subscription prices. All prices are subject to change without notice. **POSTMASTER:** Send address changes to *Critical Care Nursing Clinics of North America*, Elsevier Health Sciences Division, Subscription Customer Service, 3251 Riverport Lane, Maryland Heights, MO 63043. **Customer Service: 1-800-654-2452 (US and Canada); 314-447-8871 (outside US and Canada). Fax: 314-447-8029. E-mail:** JournalsCustomerService-usa@elsevier.com **(for print support) and** JournalsOnlineSupport-usa@elsevier.com **(for online support).**

Reprints. For copies of 100 or more of articles in this publication, please contact the Commercial Reprints Department, Elsevier Inc., 360 Park Avenue South, New York, New York, 10010-1710; Tel.: 212-633-3874, Fax: 212-633-3820, and E-mail: reprints@elsevier.com.

Critical Care Nursing Clinics of North America is covered in *MEDLINE/PubMed (Index Medicus), International Nursing Index, Nursing Citation Index, Cumulative Index to Nursing and Allied Health Literature, and RNdex Top 100.*

Contributors

CONSULTING EDITOR

DEBORAH GARBEE, PhD, APRN, ACNS-BC, FCNS
Associate Dean for Professional Practice, Community Service and Advanced Nursing Practice, Professor of Clinical Nursing, Louisiana State University Health Sciences Center New Orleans School of Nursing, Louisiana, New Orleans

EDITOR

NICOLE JUDICE JONES, MN, APRN, ACNS-BC, CV-BC, CCNS, CHFN, AACC
Clinical Nurse Specialist, Heart Failure and Structural Heart, East Jefferson General Hospital, Metairie, Louisiana, USA

AUTHORS

NASSIM ADHAMI, PhD
School of Nursing, University of British Columbia, Centre for Heart Valve Innovation, St. Paul's Hospital, Vancouver, British Columbia, Canada

WILLIAM SHANE ARRINGTON, BMSc, CNMT
Emory Healthcare, Atlanta, Georgia, USA

KELBY BIVEN, PA-C
Emory Healthcare, Atlanta, Georgia, USA

NINA BOUTTE, RN
Associate Degree in Nursing, RN-to-BSN Student, Nurse Residency Graduate and Clinical Nurse, Cardiac Telemetry Unit, East Jefferson General Hospital, Metairie, Louisiana, USA

THOMAS BROWN, BSN, RN
Emory Healthcare, Atlanta, Georgia, USA

BETH TOWERY DAVIDSON, DNP, ACNP, CHFN, FHFSA
Adjunct Faculty, Vanderbilt University School of Nursing, Director, HF Disease Management Program Centennial Heart, LLC, TriStar Centennial Medical Center, Nashville, Tennessee, USA

MARJO DE RONDE-TILLMANS, BSc
Department of Cardiology, Thoraxcenter, Erasmus University Medical Center, Rotterdam, the Netherlands

EMILY DONOVAN, NP-C
Atlanta, Georgia, USA

SABRINA DUNHAM, PharmD, BCPS, BCCP
Cardiovascular Clinical Pharmacy Specialist, Centennial Heart, LLC, TriStar Centennial Medical Center, Nashville, Tennessee, USA

JEANETTE GASTON, MSN, FNP-C
Emory Healthcare, Atlanta, Georgia, USA

MORGAN HARRISON, RN, BSN
Emory Healthcare, Atlanta, Georgia, USA

LARA S. HERNANDEZ, DNP, APRN, FNP-C
Nurse Practitioner, East Jefferson General Hospital Heart Failure Clinic, Metairie, Louisiana, USA

KENYA HESTER, APRN, MSN, CCNS, ACNS-BC
Emory Healthcare, Atlanta, Georgia, USA

MARY HIGGINS, MSN, APRN, AG-CNS
Emory Healthcare, Atlanta, Georgia, USA

BETTINA HØJBERG KIRK, MSN
Department of Cardiology, 3153 The Heart Center, Rigshospitalet Copenhagen University Hospital, Copenhagen, Denmark

VICTORIA FACQUET JOHNSON, MSN, RN, PCCN
Director of Stepdown ICU and CCU, Traction Department, East Jefferson General Hospital, Metairie, Louisiana, USA

EMILY JONES, RN, BSN
Emory Healthcare, Atlanta, Georgia, USA

NICOLE JUDICE JONES, MN, APRN, ACNS-BC, CV-BC, CCNS, CHFN, AACC
Clinical Nurse Specialist, Heart Failure and Structural Heart, East Jefferson General Hospital, Metairie, Louisiana, USA

LOUISA KALINKE, NP-C
Emory Healthcare, Atlanta, Georgia, USA

PATRICIA A. KEEGAN, DNP, NP-C, FACC
Emory Healthcare, Atlanta, Georgia, USA

SANDRA B. LAUCK, PhD
School of Nursing, University of British Columbia Centre for Heart Valve Innovation, St. Paul's Hospital Vancouver, British Columbia, Canada

JENNIFER M. MANNING, DNS, ACNS-BC, CNE
Associate Dean for Undergraduate Programs and Clinical Researcher, Louisiana State University, Health New Orleans School of Nursing, LCMC Health East Jefferson General Hospital, New Orleans, Louisiana, USA

PREETHY MATHEW, NP-C
Emory Healthcare, Atlanta, Georgia, USA

PAM MATTIO, BSN, RN, CEN, CPHQ
Clinical Quality Analyst, LCMC Health East Jefferson General Hospital, New Orleans, Louisiana, USA

GEMMA McCALMONT, MSc
James Cook University Hospital, Middlesbrough, United Kingdom

RAE MITCHELL, RN, MSN, VA-BC
Emory Healthcare, Atlanta, Georgia, USA

STACEY MOLDTHAN, RN, CHFN
Cardiac Rehab Nurse, Cardiac Rehab Department, East Jefferson General Hospital, Metairie, Louisiana, USA

CECILIA MORTORANO, MSN, RN, NEA-BC
Emory Healthcare, Atlanta, Georgia, USA

NIAMAN NAZIR, MD, MPH
Department of Population Health, Research Associate Professor, Kansas University Medical Center, Kansas City, Kansas, USA

PATRICIA O'LEARY, BSN, RN-BC
Cardiac Rehab Nurse, Cardiac Rehab Department, East Jefferson General Hospital, Metairie, Louisiana, USA

GINA M. PEEK, MSN, APRN
Department of Nursing, Associate Professor, Emporia State University, Emporia, Kansas, USA

KRYSTAL RAPHAEL, MSN, RN, CMSRN
Manager of Oncology Acute Care, Wound and Ostomy Care, Diabetes Management, East Jefferson General Hospital, Metairie, Louisiana, USA

KATHERINE M. REEDER, PhD, RN, FAHA
Adjunct Faculty Wilkes University, Passan School of Nursing, Cape Coral, Florida, USA

ANA RICHARD, LCSW
Master of Social Work, East Jefferson General Hospital, Social Work, including Heart Failure Unit, Metairie, Louisiana, USA

KIMBERLY SANDERS, RN
Associate Degree in Nursing, Nurse Residency Graduate and Clinical Nurse, Cardiac Telemetry Unit, East Jefferson General Hospital, Metairie, Louisiana, USA

AMANDA SMITH, DNP
Hamilton Health Sciences, Hamilton, Ontario, Canada

ANGELA SPAHR, BS, RDMS, RDCS
Emory Healthcare, Atlanta, Georgia, USA

CHRISTINE STONEMAN, RN, MSN, CNML, RT(R)
Emory Healthcare, Atlanta, Georgia, USA

CANDICE WAGUESPACK, BSN, RN, CHFN
Clinical Nurse, New Graduate Preceptor, Nurse Resident Mentor, Cardiac Telemetry Unit, East Jefferson General Hospital, Metairie, Louisiana, USA

LINDA L. WICK, MSN, APRN, CHFN
Fairview Health Services, President, American Association of Heart Failure Nurses, Minneapolis, Minnesota, USA

FIONA WINTERBOTTOM, DNP, MSN, APRN, ACNS-BC, ACHPN, CCRN
Advanced Practice Provider, Ochsner Health, Pulmonary Critical Care, New Orleans, Louisiana, USA

STEFFEN WUNDRAM, BSC
Universitätsklinikum, Kiel, Germany

Contents

Heart failure is a common, serious condition associated with frequent exacerbations and hospitalizations. Preventable causes of more than 70% of heart failure hospitalizations are attributable to ineffective heart failure self-care, including symptom recognition and interpretation, and delayed symptom reporting and treatment seeking. The social context in which illness symptoms occur is an important aspect of symptom self-management. Self-initiated medical and nonmedical treatments for symptom relief and engaging in lay consultations with persons in social networks for symptom evaluation are common. This article highlights socially delineated aspects of symptom self-management leading to hospitalization, many of which are amenable to nursing intervention.

Despite advances in heart failure therapies with proven positive outcomes, treatment gaps in clinical practice persist and heart failure morbidity and mortality remain high. The lack of treatment intensification to evidence-based targets accounts for a significant portion of unattained treatment goals and has been characterized to involve 3 main elements: the provider initiating and titrating the medication(s), the patient themselves, and the system that serves as the gatekeeper and facilitator for health care needs. This article will examine the mechanisms and impact of these 3 factors, and present targeted initiatives to help improve patient outcomes and quality of care.

Guideline-directed medical treatment (GDMT) is the mainstay of treatment for patients with heart failure (HF). Despite compelling evidence, patient and provider adherence to these guidelines remains low. This is mostly due to the complexity of the GDMT regimen and the competing comorbid conditions. The COVID-19 pandemic has further complicated the initiation and maintenance of GDMT and overall care for patients with HF. Telemedicine will erase many of the barriers to appropriate HF care that were present before, during, and long after the COVID-19 pandemic has ended.

Many people with heart failure also have untreated depression. Because depression can lead to worse self-care and increased morbidity and mortality for patients with heart failure, identification and treatment are essential. Nurses in clinic and inpatient settings are uniquely positioned to implement depression screening and advocate for evidence-based treatment for heart failure patients with depression. Treatments may include pharmacologic therapies, cognitive behavioral therapy, exercise, including cardiac rehabilitation, and social support. Adequate screening, treatment, and education by nurses have the potential to improve self-care for heart failure patients, thus improving morbidity and mortality of this vulnerable population.

Sepsis is a syndrome that is one of the leading causes of morbidity and mortality across the world. Those with pre-existing conditions, such as heart failure, have worse outcomes. This article will discuss the guidelines for the treatment of sepsis and opportunities to enhance the care of patients with heart failure with sepsis.

During Bachelor of Science in Nursing (BSN) program education, student nurses are introduced to topics such as patient care across health care settings, health promotion, research, safety and quality, technology, and leadership in the health care system. As one of the most common diseases in the population, heart failure (HF) is covered throughout the BSN curriculum. There are various educational strategies used by nursing schools to ensure BSN students possess the necessary leadership skills and are prepared for providing HF patient care in care management settings. Strategies include active learning education delivery models, case studies, role play, and interactive games.

Hospital-acquired pressure injuries are problematic within organizations. The Centers for Medicare and Medicaid Services counts hospital-acquired pressure injuries as a patient safety event and encourages hospitals to reduce or eliminate them in part by reducing payments to the hospital. Individuals who are admitted to hospitals with acute heart failure are usually elderly with comorbidities that increase their risk of developing a pressure injury. Therefore, evidence-based protocols should be made, implemented, and analyzed by an interprofessional team to combat the development of pressure injuries to maintain the best quality of life for patients hospitalized with heart failure.

Motivational interviewing (MI) has positive effects on heart failure patient outcomes related to self-care. MI can be effectively used by the interprofessional team in the hospital and clinic settings, and it can be effective even in brief patient interactions. The spirit of MI uses collaboration, evocation, and honoring the patient's autonomy. Open-ended questions, affirmations, reflective listening, and summarization are skills used to build empathy and elicit change talk with the MI framework. Clinicians can consider obtaining feedback to improve their practice of MI techniques for enhanced efficacy in helping heart failure patients improve self-care behaviors.

TAVR

Team-based care has been recommended by numerous cardiovascular organizations involving the treatment of valvular heart disease. Utilization of the cardiovascular team (CVT) in valvular programs has been discussed but there is a paucity of data involving team roles, backgrounds, or expectations. This article will describe a single health system and the roles of the CVT involved in the transcatheter aortic valve replacement (TAVR) program.

Transcatheter aortic valve replacement (TAVR) is an established therapy for the treatment of severe aortic stenosis. The evolution of technology and procedural approaches has facilitated the development of streamlined clinical pathways to optimize patient care and improve outcomes. The revision of historical practices and the adoption of contemporary best practices throughout patients' journey from referral to discharge create opportunities to drive quality improvement. Nursing expertise and leadership are essential to recalibrate preprocedure, periprocedure, and postprocedure practice to transform the way we care for TAVR patients, achieve excellent outcomes, and promote high-performing health services for the treatment of valvular heart disease.

Implementing healthy work environment standards helps to improve the care environment for nurses and patients. These standards were used as a framework during a nurse resident-led evidence-based practice project. The transcatheter aortic valve replacement team collaborated with the nurse residents throughout the evidence-based practice project to design a fast-track patient selection checklist and give input into a care protocol for their cardiac telemetry unit.

CRITICAL CARE NURSING
CLINICS OF NORTH AMERICA

Preface

Perspectives on Optimizing the Care of People with Heart Failure and Transcatheter Aortic Valve Replacement

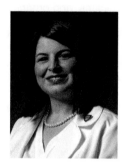

Nicole Judice Jones, MN, APRN, ACNS-BC, CV-BC, CCNS, CHFN, AACC
Editor

As a nursing profession and in collaboration with our interprofessional team colleagues, nurses have access to a wealth of clinical guidelines, consensus statements, and research evidence about how to best care for patients with heart failure. Our patient education resources are endless. Why is care not optimized for everyone? New perspectives may help us partner with our patients and colleagues to improve care through better understanding. Appreciating the beliefs of a heart failure patient, his family, and other influential individuals may help to close gaps in self-care. Several factors impact clinical inertia and incomplete optimization of guideline-directed medical therapy (GDMT), but strategies to overcome the barriers are described. Meeting our heart failure patients where they are during the COVID-19 pandemic presents unique challenges but also silver linings and progress in implementing GDMT through telemedicine. Screening for and treating depression in heart failure patients is often overlooked, although necessary for efficacious self-care. Treating heart failure patients with sepsis requires expertise and teamwork. Managing care of heart failure patients requires interactive educational preparation in population health management and clinical leadership. Prevention of pressure injury in hospitalized patients decreases morbidity and mortality, and peer feedback may enhance implementation of evidence-based strategies. Implementing motivational interviewing strategies for heart failure patients may help to elucidate the patient's personal motivations and provide a new direction to partner together to meet mutual goals for self-care.

Crit Care Nurs Clin N Am 34 (2022) xiii–xiv
https://doi.org/10.1016/j.cnc.2022.02.001
0899-5885/22/© 2022 Published by Elsevier Inc.

ccnursing.theclinics.com

There is overlap between heart failure and transcatheter aortic valve replacement (TAVR), as many patients with severe aortic stenosis present with signs and symptoms of heart failure. TAVR care is also dependent on a high-functioning team. Performance improvement and care optimization are best achieved through collaboration and teamwork. Nurses are well suited for many leadership and care coordination roles for TAVR patients, and nurse residents can be incorporated into and lead evidence-based practice changes with support and a focus on a healthy work environment.

Nurses assess patients as unique individuals, taking into account behavioral and social influences in planning and personalizing care. As clinicians who value evidence-based care, nurses are well positioned to combine the best guidelines and research evidence with fresh perspectives and individualized tools to partner for optimal care and outcomes for patients, clinicians, and organizations.

Nicole Judice Jones, MN, APRN, ACNS-BC, CV-BC, CCNS, CHFN, AACC
Heart Failure and Structural Heart
East Jefferson General Hospital
4200 Houma Boulevard
2 East, 2nd Floor
Metairie, LA 70006, USA

E-mail address:
nicole.jones4@lcmchealth.org

Heart Failure

Prehospitalization Symptom Perceptions, Lay Consultations, and Treatment-Seeking for Acute Decompensating Heart Failure: Implications for Nursing Practice

Katherine M. Reeder, PhD, RN, FAHA[a],*, Gina M. Peek, MSN, APRN[b],
Niaman Nazir, MD, MPH[c]

KEYWORDS

- Heart failure • Signs and symptoms • Perceptions • Consultations
- Self-management • Nursing care

KEY POINTS

- Symptom perceptions, including symptom recognition, interpretation, and attribution are variable among patients regardless of the length of time patients have lived with heart failure and whether patients have experienced previous HF hospitalizations.
- Engaging with persons from patients' social networks for symptom evaluation (ie, lay consultations) is common in heart failure symptom self-management.
- Prompt symptom reporting and treatment seeking soon after symptom onset is paramount for receiving timely professional health care treatments and avoiding potentially preventable hospitalizations.

INTRODUCTION AND BACKGROUND
Epidemiologic Burden of Heart Failure

Despite advances in prevention and treatment modalities, heart failure (HF) has remained a major public health problem in the United States and globally for nearly 30 years. HF affects more than 6.0 million Americans; by 2030, the prevalence of HF is estimated to increase by 46%.[1] HF is the primary discharge diagnosis for roughly

[a] Wilkes University, Passan School of Nursing, 84 West South Street, Wilkes-Barre, PA 18766, USA; [b] Department of Nursing, Emporia State University, Campus Box 4043, Cora Miller Hall, 206C, Emporia, KS 66801, USA; [c] Department of Population Health, Kansas University Medical Center, Mail Stop 1008, 3901 Rainbow Boulevard. Kansas City, KS 66160, USA
* Corresponding author.
E-mail addresses: kcmvrk@yahoo.com; katherine.reeder@wilkes.edu

Crit Care Nurs Clin N Am 34 (2022) 129–140
https://doi.org/10.1016/j.cnc.2022.02.002
0899-5885/22/© 2022 Elsevier Inc. All rights reserved.

1.0 million and the secondary discharge diagnosis for 2.0 million hospitalizations annually.[2] Mortality rates and the level of health care resource use for patients with HF are among the highest associated with any medical condition.[2] Patients admitted to the hospital with HF have a 20% to 30% risk of death within 1 year.[2] HF makes up nearly 2% of the total US health care budget, of which more than one-half accounts for HF inpatient hospital stays.[2]

Disparities in HF persist, with Black persons having the greatest risk of developing HF and a higher risk of hospitalization and death compared with Hispanic, White non-Hispanic, and Chinese American persons.[1,3–5] In addition, people who live in rural communities in the Western, Midwestern, and Southern regions of the United States have a higher risk of death during HF hospitalization compared with their urban counterparts, regardless of ethnic background.[1] Rates of HF hospital readmission are higher in patients previously hospitalized for HF, and as few as one-tenth of eligible patients receive cardiac rehabilitation referral at discharge from HF hospitalization.[1] Individual social determinants of health, such as age, race, education, cognitive status, health literacy, and social support, are associated with mortality after a hospitalization for HF, indicating these factors might be independent markers of vulnerability after hospital discharge. In a recent study aligned with the Healthy People 2020 goals, 690 Medicare patients who had even one of the social determinants of health (ie, being Black, having no one to care for you when ill, living in a health provider shortage area, living in a rural area) had nearly 3 times the risk of death within 90 days after discharge from an HF hospitalization compared with patients with no social determinants of health risk factors.[6] These figures are alarming, given hospitalization alone is a risk factor for increased morbidity and premature death in patients with HF.[7]

Although much of the research and clinical practice to date has focused on mechanistic pathways of HF (eg, HF with reduced ejection fraction; HF with preserved ejection fraction), the identification of risk factors and preventive strategies, and medical treatments for HF (eg, novel medications, cardiac resynchronization therapy, implantable cardiac defibrillator, left ventricular assist device, and heart transplant surgery), attention to the social determinants of health, including the context in which symptoms occur, is lacking.[8] Using an HF self-management framework (**Fig. 1**), this article highlights symptom-related activities patients engage in, as part of their daily lives before being hospitalized for acute decompensated HF, including symptom perceptions, interactions with others from their social networks about symptoms (ie, lay consultations), self-initiated strategies used for symptom relief, and the timeliness in which patients report symptoms to health care providers and seek professional care for symptoms.

Symptom Perceptions

Ineffective self-care is attributable to more than one-half of preventable HF hospitalizations.[9–11] Self-care is defined as a real-world, natural process of decision-making by which individuals choose behaviors to maintain physiologic stability, monitor for changes in stability, and manage changes in stability by evaluating physiologic changes, taking action to treat changes, and then assessing the outcome of or response to those actions.[11] The cornerstone of HF self-care is symptom self-management, which depends on individuals being able to expeditiously recognize, interpret, and report worsening HF symptoms to health care providers.[12] Initially, however, worsening HF symptoms are often vague and can wax and wane over time, making it difficult to recognize and interpret subtle somatic changes of an impending HF exacerbation episode.[13] In addition, symptoms are frequently misattributed to other conditions, changes in prescription medications, diet or exercise routines, or even

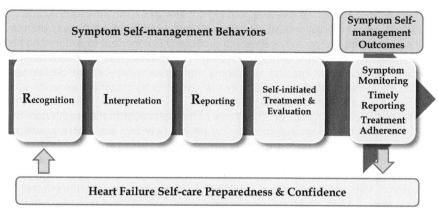

Fig. 1. HF Symptom self-management framework.

aging.[1,13,14] For example, many patients report vague feelings that something is "just not quite right," or they "feel different from normal" before symptom onset, but are unable to name any particular symptoms, which indicates patients might experience prodromal symptoms where they sense potential warning signs of physiologic instability, but these changes have not yet manifested into detectable symptoms.[14,15]

In a previous study, more than 93% of patients did not realize before being hospitalized that their symptoms were related to acute decompensated HF; more than 40% of patients thought their symptoms were due to recent changes in their self-care regimens (ie, diet, medications, weight, sleep, or exercise).[14] Other patient attributions for symptoms included (1) recent hospitalization, (2) change in usual routine, (3) increased fluid intake, (4) lack of motivation, (5) yard work, (6) drastic weather changes, or (7) unstable housing. Once patients were able to clearly detect and name their symptoms, dyspnea, fatigue, and edema were identified as the symptoms that ultimately led to their hospitalization. Most often, by the time patients experienced significant dyspnea, fatigue, and/or edema, hospitalization was unavoidable.

Symptom misperception is a pervasive problem for patients with HF and is often due to patients being discharged from the hospital with unresolved symptoms, which can hinder effective self-management. Patients discharged from the hospital with unresolved symptoms have difficulties in not only discerning changes in unresolved symptoms, but also in detecting new symptoms, adding to the complexity and burden of HF symptom self-management.[14,16] Early and consistent postdischarge nursing care focused on HF symptom self-management strategies for resolving symptoms throughout the postacute period after hospital discharge might add an extra layer of transitional support for patients who self-manage their symptoms.

Lay Consultations in Symptom Evaluation

Engaging in lay consultations (ie, social interactions with persons in one's social network for symptom evaluation) is quite common and has been shown to influence patients' understanding of symptoms and their decision-making about what to do for symptoms.[14,17–20] Patients who experience illness-related symptoms often engage in an array of self-care activities, including lay consultations and self-initiated treatments, such as over-the-counter medications and other remedies before, after, or in lieu of seeking professional health care. Engaging in self-care activities for commonly occurring nonfatal illness symptoms among otherwise healthy adults is not only appropriate, but encouraged before seeking professional care; however, such is not the case for persons living with HF. Because decision-making about illness symptoms is often a complex and socially delineated process, it is important to understand how people form cognitive representations (eg, internal mental symbols that represent the external reality) of their cardiac symptoms and make health-related decisions to develop interventions that will effectively prevent HF hospitalization, expedite treatment seeking, and optimize health outcomes.

As most symptoms initially occur outside of the domain of formal health care systems, it is important to understand how lay referral networks and, more specifically lay consultations, influence symptom perceptions and treatment-seeking decision-making among patients experiencing worsening symptoms of HF. Lay referral networks can provide a venue for social comparison and information exchange.[21] Patients experiencing cardiac symptoms may consult others in their lay referral network before seeking professional care, especially if they are uncertain about the meaning of their symptoms. Even in the face of uncertainty, however, most people formulate an initial explanation of their symptoms. If patients' initial common sense explanations are validated by others in their lay referral network, the level of uncertainty about their symptoms is decreased.[22] Because members of one's lay referral network frequently offer their own interpretations of symptoms, they are in a unique position to influence perceptions of symptoms, common sense explanations of symptoms, and not only whether to seek professional care for symptoms, but also how soon that care is sought. Thus, lay consultations may have a positive, as well as a negative, impact on symptom perceptions and the timeliness in which treatment for symptoms is sought.[23]

To investigate the role of lay consultations in symptom evaluation and treatment-seeking behavior among persons who experienced an acute myocardial infarction (AMI), interview data from both patients who had an AMI and the lay consultant with whom they consulted foremost were analyzed.[17] There was virtually no agreement between patients with AMI and their lay consultants on symptoms, perceptions of potential causes of symptoms (ie, symptom attributions), and advice on what to do about symptoms. When lay consultants thought patients who had an AMI experienced typical symptoms of AMI (crushing chest pain; jaw, neck, or arm pain), they were significantly more likely to attribute symptoms to cardiac causes than when patients, themselves, expressed they experienced typical AMI symptoms. An incongruent pattern between symptom attributions and advice was also observed in that, neither patients' nor lay consultants' symptom perceptions predicted lay consultants' advice on what to do about symptoms. And, neither lay consultants' symptom attributions nor their advice predicted the timeliness in which patients sought treatment. In these patients and lay consultants, symptom perceptions and attributions did not influence the timeliness of seeking treatment; what persons who experienced AMI recollected as the advice that was given to them by lay consultants significantly prolonged delay in seeking treatment, whereas the actual advice given by lay consultants had no discernible impact on the timeliness of seeking treatment.

In a more recent study on HF symptom self-management, more than 70% of the lay consultants attributed patients' symptoms to a heart problem, followed by lung problems and diabetes.[24] Interestingly, patients received advice about what to do for symptoms more often than they received symptom attributions from lay consultants; thus, even when lay consultants did not offer thoughts on symptom causes, they offered advice on what to do about symptoms. Although more than 95% of lay consultants' advice was to seek medical care, the timeliness of seeking professional care for symptoms was overall suboptimal (2 hours to 2 weeks). Men engaged in lay consultations more frequently than women and most often consulted with their spouse, whereas women most often consulted with their adult children.

The sociocultural context in which illness symptoms occur is an important concern for nursing because expeditious care-seeking behavior for symptoms can translate into improved clinical outcomes. Results of these studies highlight some of the difficulties in teasing out the role of lay consultations before an HF hospitalization and warrants further attention as a potentially influential aspect of symptom self-management. Nursing interventions that effectively address social influence processes, such as lay consultations in symptom self-management are needed.

Timeliness of Seeking Treatment for Symptoms

Although few studies have focused on how older adults cope with symptoms in their day-to-day lives, it is likely that self-initiated care, including nonmedical treatments are prevalent.[25] Although specific self-initiated treatments might be appropriate and even encouraged by health care providers as an integral part of patients' symptom self-management, the time it takes patients to recognize and interpret symptoms of worsening HF and engage in self-initiated strategies to relieve symptoms and then assess whether treatments improved symptoms adds to delays in receiving timely professional care and avoiding potentially preventable hospitalizations. In a previous study, 40% of patients reported using both medical and nonmedical self-initiated strategies aimed at relieving symptoms.[14] Self-medication was the most common strategy used for symptom relief; however, there was wide variation in the medications used by patients and included the use of furosemide (Lasix), nitroglycerin, prescription pain medication, metformin, aspirin, oxygen, and breathing treatments. Raising the head of the bed, resting, walking, and diet changes were some of the nonmedical strategies used for symptom relief.

Although the literature is replete with studies on treatment-seeking delay in HF, research on symptom reporting, as a component of total treatment-seeking delay times, is sparse. Treatment-seeking delay, or prehospital delay, has been defined as the duration between symptom onset and hospital arrival; however, in nursing studies, prehospital delay times were often defined as the time between symptom onset and patients' decision to seek professional care for symptoms to account for transit times between patients' locations (eg, home) and presenting hospitals.[14,26] Findings to date indicate patients with HF who are men, younger, and Black, as well as those who have multiple presenting symptoms, dyspnea and edema, higher symptom distress, no prior history of HF, symptom onset during early morning hours (midnight to 6:00 AM), worse New York Heart Association functional status, and gradual symptom onset or being cared for by a primary care physician (vs a cardiologist) delay seeking treatment for their HF symptoms than patients without these characteristics.[27-33] However, social aspects of symptom self-management described in this article (eg, symptom recognition, interpretation and reporting, as well as self-initiated treatments used and engagement in lay consultations) are virtually absent from the literature.

The timeliness of seeking care, including prehospital delay for cardiac symptoms, has received a great deal of attention in the health-related literature. However, few studies have attempted to examine the prehospitalization timeline of events that occur relative to symptom self-management during the symptomatic period. For example, Reeder and colleagues[14] found that, after symptom onset and before being hospitalized for acute decompensated HF, many patients felt they needed to contact their health care provider or go to the hospital, but few patients actually did so. When patients were asked what made them think they needed to seek treatment for their symptoms, salient signs and symptoms, such as shortness of breath, swelling, weight gain, irregular heartbeat, fatigue, and chest pain were reported, all indicative of worsening symptoms of HF that commonly result in hospitalization.[14] When asked about the timeliness of symptom reporting and treatment seeking, patients said when they contacted their health care provider, it took time for their health care provider to call them back, time to be evaluated in the outpatient clinic by their health care provider if seen at the clinic, as well as time to be seen in the emergency department or admitted to the hospital (**Fig. 2**).[14]

More than one-third of the patients attempted to contact their health care provider during the symptomatic period from 2 weeks up to 2 days before hospitalization.[14] Patients who contacted their health care provider waited for a callback for 15 minutes to 24 hours. The median time between initial patient contact with their health care provider and being seen in the emergency department or admitted to the hospital was 6 hours, with a range from 30 minutes to 15 days. Patients who were evaluated by their health care provider in the outpatient setting before hospitalization waited 10 minutes to 37 days for their clinic appointment. The median time between a patient's clinic visit and hospitalization was 2 hours, with a range of 20 minutes to 14 days. This timeline of prehospital HF self-management events demonstrates unnecessary delay times in every component of prehospital delay explored.

The time it takes patients to recognize and interpret worsening symptoms of HF, consult with others from their lay referral network about symptoms, engage in self-initiated treatments for symptom relief, and decide to seek professional care can significantly delay patients from receiving effective timely treatments, lengthen

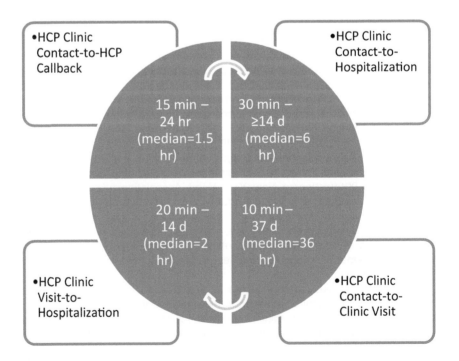

*HCP = Healthcare Provider

Fig. 2. Pre-hospitalization symptom reporting action behavior timelines .

inpatient hospital stays, increase morbidity and mortality, prolong recovery, and hinder the effectiveness of HF symptom self-management in the postdischarge environment.

DISCUSSION

Taken together, previous studies indicate a variety of social factors can significantly influence symptom perception, interpretation, attribution, and treatment-seeking decision-making. Misattribution of symptoms is frequent among patients with HF, especially elderly patients who have multiple conditions. Multimorbidity among aging populations is common and adds to the complexity of medical treatment and self-care, including HF symptom self-management.

Although patient recall of information shared by health care providers is important for implementing provider-directed HF recommendations to enhance health and prevent worsening symptoms and future exacerbations, patient recall of professional advice about symptom self-management depends on patients being able to recognize, interpret, and attribute their symptoms to HF in a timely manner. As demonstrated by Reeder and colleagues[14] in exploring components of the prehospital symptomatic period, patients did not recognize and interpret their symptoms early on as being attributable to HF, regardless of having previously received an HF diagnosis and patient education. Thus, it is plausible that patients are unable to act on patient education instructions and professional advice previously received until symptoms reach a critical point of being clearly detected and named. The Think of Your Heart First – TYHF initiative is a research-based patient education, easy-to-remember acronym (similar to the commonly used "Thank goodness it's Friday – TGIF" acronym) developed to encourage patients to think of their heart first, regardless of the symptoms they experience as part of an effort to expedite treatment and reduce hospitalizations. The TYHF initiative grew out of recurrent study findings of low levels of symptom recognition, interpretation, and reporting, as well as prolonged delays in seeking treatment for worsening symptoms of HF.

Symptom attributions are quite variable and could influence the type and frequency of strategies used for symptom relief. Differences in strategies patients use to relieve symptoms are typical, which might be, in part, attributable to the socialization of lifelong patterns of illness perceptions and self-initiated treatment decision-making.[14] Self-initiated medical and nonmedical treatments, although common, often draw questions about safety and quality. For example, metformin is commonly prescribed as a once daily medication for diabetes, with more recent use in HF; however, taking extra doses of metformin as a self-initiated medical treatment for worsening symptoms of HF could be dangerous for patients and result in untoward outcomes.

The postdischarge environment contributes to the effectiveness of HF self-care. For example, the stability of patients' community and more specifically, home environment can significantly impact HF self-care and the risk for hospitalization.[34,35] The hospital environment is organized systematically, with nursing care departments consisting of homogeneous patient groups where standard guideline-based approaches to care are the norm. In contrast, the postdischarge environment is heterogenous and by nature, individually unique (**Table 1**).[14] Thus, nursing interventions aimed at facilitating HF self-care after hospital discharge must be adapted to meet individual patient needs within the context of their environment.

Engaging in social interactions about symptoms in chronic illness is common.[18] Previous studies demonstrate that discussing symptoms with others (ie, lay consultation) is an important strategy for patients trying to interpret their symptoms, as evidenced by nearly 80% of patients who sought advice from others. Interestingly, only 71% of lay consultants attributed patients' symptoms to cardiac causes; however, an overwhelming majority (95%) advised patients to seek professional care.[24] Although nearly all of the patients said they took the advice of others to seek medical care for symptoms, nearly 20% of patients delayed 5 days or more to actively seek medical care.

Research that examines whether uncertainty about symptoms leads patients to interact with and seek advice from other lay persons about symptoms before seeking professional care, how lay consultants perceive symptoms and give advice about what to do for symptoms, and whether dyads of patients and lay consultants can expedite symptom reporting and treatment-seeking behavior is needed. Findings from studies included in this article highlight the complexities of teasing out the contributions of lay consultations on symptom interpretation and treatment-seeking behavior and underscore the need for including key lay consultants (eg, spouses/domestic partners, adult children, other informal caregivers) in HF self-management patient education and hospital-to-home transitional programs of care.

The timeliness of reporting symptoms to health care providers, if reported at all, is variable. Despite more than one-half of patients feeling the need to contact their health care provider or go to the hospital when symptoms began, few patients actually contacted their health care provider before hospital admission.[24] Worth noting is that nearly one-half of the patients who contacted their health care provider before hospitalization did so from 2 to more than 14 days after symptom onset. Thus, further research is warranted on the impact of early reporting of symptoms to health care providers on hospitalization, clinical outcomes, and health care costs.

The contributions of health care provider response times to patients on the timeliness of receiving effective timely HF treatments is noteworthy. When patients contact health care providers, messages are left most often with clinic receptionists who, in turn, give patients' messages to physicians or clinic nurses while patients wait for a call back, either from the nurse or physician. Although the median response time to patients by health care providers was 1 to 1.5 hours, some patients waited up to 24 hours during nonweekend days. The time between contacting health care providers and being seen in the emergency department or admitted to the hospital was quite variable, with a median of 6 hours and upwards of more than 2 weeks. Only one-half of the patients who contacted their health care provider were evaluated during a clinic visit before hospitalization, with wait times for clinic appointments ranging from a few minutes up to more than 6 weeks. From the clinic visit, wait times to hospitalization ranged from less than 30 minutes to up to 2 weeks.

Medical treatments for acutely decompensating HF are time dependent, meaning that the early treatment of patients with evolving symptoms can potentially prevent HF hospitalization and shorten hospital length of stay once patients are admitted to

Table 1	
Characteristics of contexts of HF care: Hospital ≠ home	
Hospital	**Home**
Other managed	Self-managed
Immediate to timely symptom response by nurses and other health care providers	Symptom response delays by patients, health care providers, and health care system
Timely, guideline-based professional health care treatments	Timely and/or untimely and medical and/or nonmedical self-initiated treatments
Standardized care environment	Individually unique care environment

the hospital. Further research is warranted that examines specific components of treatment-seeking delays, including the timeliness of symptom recognition and interpretation and the context in which symptoms occur and are reported to health care providers, as well as the context in which health care providers respond and act on patient reports. Nursing interventions are needed that include navigation triggers within the health care system for patients who have HF such that, when patients contact their health care provider, an HF protocol is initiated for making same-day appointments to assess and treat patients in the outpatient setting and, if needed, directly admit patients to hospital nursing departments for care of patients with HF to avoid long delays in the emergency department.

CLINICS CARE POINTS

- Assessing symptom experiences from symptom onset through the course of treatment seeking can reveal important information for addressing in nursing interventions that would otherwise remain obscure For example, delays in symptom interpretation and seeking treatment, as well as self-initiated medical and nonmedical strategies used to relieve symptoms are areas of self-care nurses can address in HF self-care interventions. To span the context of self-care outside of the purview of formal health care systems, nurses can uniquely address HF self-care in the postdischarge environment.

- Symptom attributions are especially problematic for patients, as evidenced by patient attributions to conditions, activities, and treatments other than HF. Approaches such as the Think of Your Heart First – TYHF initiative can help patients to report symptom experiences early after symptom onset or even, during the presymptom prodromal period. By doing so, patients can be evaluated and possibly, treated in the outpatient setting, avoiding potentially preventable hospitalizations. To achieve this goal, mechanisms must be in place for initiating HF protocols from the intake call by clinic receptionists to initial in-person nursing assessments to evaluation and activation of a medical treatment plan by physicians.

- Engaging in lay consultations for symptom evaluation can expedite or delay treatment-seeking behavior. Investigators most often found that taking time to consult with others in patients' lay referral network results in unnecessary treatment delays. Most often, however, patients engage in lay consultations with spouses and adult children, all of whom are integral to patients' HF self-care and might just be the ones who ultimately convince patients to seek professional care for symptoms. Including key lay consultants in the HF self-care can optimize self-care outcomes, including timely treatment seeking.

- Patients discharged from the HF hospitalizations often have unresolved symptoms and even new symptoms related to HF treatments during hospitalization that can be confusing for patients to self-manage in the immediate, postacute period. In addition to feeling weak and sometimes, exhausted, pets needing care, lack of grocery items, piled up mail and bills to pay, yard work needing to be completed, and house cleaning and laundry needs are just a few of the reasons patients report for unfilled prescriptions and implementing daily weights, exercise, and diet changes during follow-up calls and visits. Many patients discharged from an HF hospitalization need tangible support during the postacute period, so they can rest and focus on implementing their HF self-care discharge instructions.

ACKNOWLEDGMENTS

The authors thank Nancy O'Brien, Director and Maureen Gullen, Library Associate of the Health Sciences Library at UnityPoint in Des Moines, Iowa for their constant support in the development and writing of this manuscript.

DISCLOSURE

Research reported in this publication was supported by the National Institute of Nursing Research of the National Institutes of Health under award numbers R00NR012217. The content is solely the responsibility of the authors and does not necessarily represent the official views of the National Institutes of Health or the National Institute of Nursing Research.

CONFLICTS OF INTEREST

The authors have no conflicts of interest to disclose.

REFERENCES

1. Virani SS, Alonso A, Aparicio HJ, et al, On behalf of the American Heart Association Council on Epidemiology and Prevention Statistics Committee and Stroke. Statistics Subcommittee. Heart disease and stroke statistics—2021 update: a report from the American Heart Association. Circulation 2021;143:e254–743.
2. Hollenberg SM, Warner Stevenson L, Ahmad T, et al. 2019 ACC expert consensus decision pathway on risk assessment, management, and clinical trajectory of patients hospitalized with heart failure: a report of the American College of Cardiology Solution Set Oversight Committee. J Am Coll Cardiol 2019;74: 1966–2011.
3. Nayak A, Hicks AJ, Morris AA. Understanding the complexity of heart failure risk and treatment in black patients. Circ Heart Fail 2020;13(8):e007264.
4. Roger VL. Epidemiology of heart failure: a contemporary perspective. Circ Res 2021;128:1421–34.
5. Cockerham WC, Hamby BW, Oates GR. The social determinants of chronic disease. Am J Prev Med 2017;52(1 Suppl 1):S5–12. https://doi.org/10.1016/j.amepre.2016.09.010.
6. Sterling MR, Bryan Ringel J, Pinheiro LC, et al. Social determinants of health and 90-day mortality after hospitalization for heart failure in the REGARDS study. J Am Heart Assoc 2020;9:e014836.
7. Will JC, Valderrama AL, Yoon PW. Preventable hospitalizations for congestive heart failure: establishing a baseline to monitor trends and disparities. Prev Chronic Dis 2012;9:110260.
8. Yancy CW, Jessup M, Bozkurt B, et al. 2013 ACCF/AHA guideline for the management of heart failure: a report of the American college of cardiology foundation/American heart association task force on practice guidelines. J Am Coll Cardiol 2013;62(16):e147–239.
9. Gilotra NA, Shpigel A, Okwuosa IS, et al. Patients commonly believe their heart failure hospitalizations are preventable and identify worsening heart failure, non-adherence, and a knowledge gap as reasons for admission. J Card Fail 2017; 23(3):252–6.
10. Fonarow GC, Abraham WT, Albert NM, et al. Factors identified as precipitating hospital admissions for heart failure and clinical outcomes: findings from OPTI-MIZE-HF. Arch Intern Med 2008;168(8):847–54.
11. Riegel B, Moser DK, Anker SD, et al, On behalf of the American Heart Association Council on Cardiovascular Nursing, Council on Clinical Cardiology, Council on Nutrition, Physical Activity, and Metabolism, and Interdisciplinary Council on Quality of Care and Outcomes Research. State of the science: promoting self-

care in persons with heart failure: a scientific statement from the American Heart Association. Circulation 2009;120:1141–63.

12. Friedman MM, Quinn JR. Heart failure patients' time, symptoms, and actions before a hospital admission. J Cardiovasc Nurs 2008;23(6):506–12.

13. Martin R, Lemos K, Rothrock N, et al. Gender disparities in common sense models in illness among myocardial infarction victims. Health Psychol 2004; 23(4):345–53.

14. Reeder KM, Ercole PM, Peek GM, et al. Symptom perceptions and self-care behaviors in patients who self-manage heart failure. J Cardiovasc Nurs 2015; 30(1):E1–7.

15. McLachlana S, Mansella G, Sandersb T, et al. Symptom perceptions and help-seeking behaviour prior to lung and colorectal cancer diagnoses: a qualitative study. Fam Pract 2015;32(5):568–77.

16. Bueno H, Ross JS, Wang Y, et al. Trend in length of stay and short-term outcomes among Medicare patients hospitalized for heart failure, 1993-2006. JAMA 2010; 303(21):2141–7.

17. Piamjariyakul U, Reeder KM, Wongpiriyayothar A, et al. Coaching: an innovative teaching strategy in heart failure home management. In: Henderson JP, Lawrence AD, editors. NOVA science: teaching strategies. New York: NOVA Science Publishers; 2011. p. 185–202.

18. Schoenberg NE, Amey CH, Stoller EP, et al. Lay referral patterns involved in cardiac treatment decision making among middle-aged and older adults. Gerontologist 2003;43(4):493–502.

19. Queenan JA, Glottlieb BH, Feldman-Stewart D, et al. Symptom appraisal, help seeking, and lay consultancy for symptoms of head and neck cancer. Psycho-Oncology 2018;27:286–94.

20. Sethares KA, Sosa MA, Fisher P, et al. Factors associated with delay in seeking care for acute decompensated heart failure. J Cardiovasc Nurs 2014;29(5): 429–38.

21. Suls J, Martin R, Leventhal H. Social comparison, lay referral, and the decision to seek medical care. In: Buunk BP, Gibbons FX, editors. Health, coping, and well-being: perspectives from social comparison theory. Mahwah, New Jersey: Lawrence Erlbaum Associates; 1997. p. 195–226.

22. Freidson E. Client control of medical practice. Am J Sociol 1960;65(4):374–82.

23. Alonzo AA. The impact of the family and lay others on care-seeking during life-threatening episodes of suspected coronary artery disease. Soc Sci Med 1986; 22:1297–311.

24. Reeder KM, Sims JL, Ercole PM, et al. Lay consultations in heart failure symptom evaluation. SOJ NurS Health Care 2017;3(2):1–7.

25. Hickey T, Akiyama H, Rakowski W. Daily illness characteristics and health care decisions of older people. J Appl Gerontol 1991;10(2):169–84.

26. Bunde J, Martin R. Depression and prehospital delay in the context of myocardial infarction. Psychosom Med 2006;68:51–7.

27. Evangelista LS, Dracup K, Doering LV. Racial differences in treatment-seeking delays among heart failure patients. J Card Fail 2002;8(6):381–6.

28. Goldberg RJ, Goldberg JH, Pruell S, et al. Delays in seeking medical care in hospitalized patients with decompensated heart failure. Am J Med 2008;121:212–8.

29. Jurgens CY. Somatic awareness, uncertainty, and delay in care-seeking in acute heart failure. Res Nurs Health 2006;29:74–86.

30. Patel H, Shafazand M, Schaufelberger M, et al. Reasons for seeking acute care in chronic heart failure. Eur J Heart Fail 2007;9:702–8.

31. Gravely-Witte S, Corrine Y, Jurgens CY, et al. Length of delay in seeking medical care by patients with heart failure symptoms and the role of symptom- related factors: a narrative review. Eur J Cardiovasc Nurs 2010;12:1122–9.

32. Okada A, Tsuchihashi-Makaya M, Kang JH, et al. Symptom perception, evaluation, response to symptom, and delayed care seeking in patients with acute heart failure: an observational study. J Cardiovasc Nurs 2019;34(1):36–43.

33. Altice NF, Madigan EA. Factors associated with delayed care-seeking in hospitalized patients with heart failure. Heart Lung 2012;41(3):244–54.

34. Hersh AM, Masoudi FA, Allen LA. Postdischarge environment following heart failure hospitalization: expanding the view of hospital readmission. J Am Heart Assoc 2013;2:e000116.

35. Wakefield BJ, Boren SA, Groves PA, et al. Heart failure care management programs: a review of study interventions and meta-analysis of outcomes. J Cardiovasc Nurs 2013;28(1):9–19.

The Perfect Storm
Barriers to Heart Failure Treatment Optimization

Beth Towery Davidson, DNP, ACNP, CHFN, FHFSA[a],*,
Sabrina Dunham, PharmD, BCPS, BCCP[b]

KEYWORDS

- clinical inertia • Heart failure • Treatment optimization
- Guideline-directed medical therapy

KEY POINTS

- Heart failure morbidity and mortality remain high despite advances in medical and device therapy.
- Patients with heart failure should receive guideline-directed medical therapy (GDMT) as outlined in published guidelines and consensus documents.
- Prescription and up-titration of medical therapy to target doses remain below expectations, due to multiple factors described as clinical inertia.
- Strategies to maximize GDMT in the heart failure population are warranted to address all components within the clinical inertia model, which includes provider, patient, and system factors.

INTRODUCTION

Treatment gaps in heart failure persist in clinical practice despite advances in heart failure therapies and strong guideline recommendations.[1] Globally, hospitalization and mortality remain high, with an estimated $30.7 billion cost burden in the United States (US) which is expected to double by 2030 .[2] Researchers continue to pursue newer cutting-edge therapies to recruit better outcomes, and important leaders in the field are actively ruminating how newer therapies will fit into current treatment models. Newer agents can certainly impact the landscape of heart failure by offering new mechanistic advantages or possessing characteristics that may be better tolerated in certain heart failure phenotypes. However, novel agents may also fall short of their potential as is currently being seen with standard evidence-based therapies. In 2019, the US Food and Drug Administration (FDA) approved 2 additional device

[a] Centennial Heart, LLC, TriStar Centennial Medical Center, 2400 Patterson Street, Nashville, TN 37203, USA; [b] Department of Pharmacy, TriStar Centennial Medical Center, 2300 Patterson Street, Nashville, TN 37203, USA
* Corresponding author. 6549 Westfall Drive, Nashville, TN 37221.
E-mail address: beth.davidson@hcahealthcare.com

Crit Care Nurs Clin N Am 34 (2022) 141–150
https://doi.org/10.1016/j.cnc.2022.02.003
0899-5885/22/© 2022 Elsevier Inc. All rights reserved.
ccnursing.theclinics.com

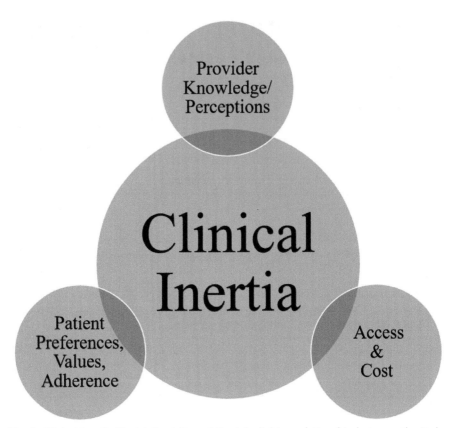

Fig. 1. Clinical Inertia Model. Depiction of the interlinking relationship between the 3 elements identified as barriers to optimal use of guideline-directed medical therapy. (*Adapted from* O'Conner's conceptual model)

therapies for heart failure. MitraClip received an expanded indication for functional mitral regurgitation and the Optimizer Smart System (cardiac contractility modulation) was approved for patients who do not meet the standard criteria for cardiac resynchronization.[3] Both device therapies require "optimal medical management," once again calling for an emphasis on baseline guideline-directed medical therapy (GDMT).[3]

CLINICAL INERTIA

Clinical inertia is defined as the lack of therapy intensification to goals based on evidence and guideline recommendations.[4] This issue has been reported extensively in chronic disease states, and heart failure is no exception.[4,5] Clinical inertia has been described to encompass 3 main factors: physician factors, patient factors, and system factors, each contributing 50%, 30%, and 20%, respectively.[4] Characterizing the underlying barriers to the optimization of guideline-directed medical therapies and developing targeted initiatives for improvement is critically important to improve patient outcomes and quality of care (**Fig.1**). In the following sections, each factor in the clinical inertia model will be examined individually, as will potential strategies to help alleviate those barriers.

PHYSICIAN/CLINICIAN/PROVIDER ROLE

Perhaps one of the most important factors that can be impacted in the clinical inertia model is that related to clinicians. Several studies, registries, and surveys conducted both nationally and internationally have overwhelmingly demonstrated the lack of pharmacotherapy intensification among providers as prescribed by the guidelines **Table 1**. IMPROVE HF (Improve the Use of Evidence-Based Heart Failure Therapies in the Outpatient Setting), a large-scale quality improvement initiative conducted in the US, collected data from 167 outpatient cardiology practices to characterize the use of standard HF therapies at the time.[6] Baseline target dosing of angiotensin-converting enzyme inhibitors (ACEI)/angiotensin II receptor blockers (ARB), beta-blocker, and mineralocorticoid receptor antagonists (MRA) in eligible patients was reported as 36.1%, 20.5%, and 74.4%, respectively.[7] At 24 months, minimal increases in number of patients at target doses were reported, with ACEI/ARB therapy at 37.9%, beta-blocker 30.3%, and MRA 78.4%.[7] Moving forward, the contemporary CHAMP-HF (Change the Management of Patients with Heart Failure) registry was a prospective observational study conducted in 150 US primary care and cardiology outpatient practices almost a decade later.[8] The angiotensin-receptor neprilysin inhibitor (ARNI) was added to the GDMT arsenal. Results revealed that 73.4% of patients were treated with ACEI/ARB/ARNI (60.5% ACEI/ARB and 13% ARNI), 67.0% with beta-blockers, and 33.4% with an MRA. Of these patients, the percentage achieving target doses were 17% (ACEI/ARB), 14% (ARNI), 28% (beta-blocker), and 77% (MRA).[8] Surprisingly, ACEI/ARB therapy had decreased over the last decade, and ARNI therapy was underutilized. Similarly, GUIDE-IT (Guiding Evidence-Based Therapy Using Biomarker Intensified Treatment in Heart Failure), a randomized multicenter trial conducted in the US and Canada, reported a mere 31% of patients reaching target ACEI/ARB doses and 15% for beta-blockers.[9]

Similar findings are echoed in European studies and registries. The BIOSTAT-CHF (Biology Study to Tailored Treatment in Chronic Heart Failure) reported achieving target dosing at 22% and 12% for ACEI/ARB and beta-blockers, respectively.[10] Likewise, a small study conducted by Diamant and colleagues in 370 patients with HF showed eligible patients at target dose for ACEI/ARB/ARNI, beta-blocker, and MRA was 29%, 32%, and 4%, respectively.[11] Other observational studies, such as the QUALIFY (QUality of Adherence to guideline recommendations for LIFe-saving treatment in heart failure) survey, ESC (European Society of Cardiology) HF Long-term registry, and the CHECK-HF (Chronisch Hartfalen ESC-richtlijn Cardiologische praktijk Kwaliteitsproject HartFalen) registry report similar findings.[12–15]

It is well-established that target dosing is related to improved morbidity and mortality outcomes.[12,16] Reasons that influenced medication titration in these studies were variable, but notably common themes exist. Reticence to up-titrate therapies was most common in more vulnerable patients, including those of advanced age, more advanced HF disease, high number of comorbidities, recent HF hospitalization, chronic kidney disease, lower systolic blood pressure, and minority status.[8,17] Certainly, not all reluctance to optimize GDMT is inappropriate, such as in the setting of intolerance or contraindicated use, and certainly clinical judgment is paramount; however, some reasons for not titrating medications to the goal are not validated by the data. Several reasons for provider reluctance to up-titrate medications have been identified in the literature and include misapplication, unfamiliarity, or disagreement with evidence-based guideline recommendations, overrating the quality of care being delivered, fear of causing clinical worsening, or "rocking the boat" when a patient seems to be "doing well" or "looks good," patient reluctance, economic feasibility, and knowledge gaps related to pharmacotherapy indication, dosing schemes, and study findings.[17–20]

Clinicians must be proficient with the patient and symptom monitoring, medication dose titration, and optimization of therapy. Unfamiliarity with target doses and personal fears that patients will not tolerate the next increment in dose contributes to the widespread failure to achieve and maintain optimal medical management.[21] Shared decision-making with an interdisciplinary team and continual medication education, coupled with other tested strategies such as the implementation of evidence-based algorithms or clinical pathways, standardized encounter forms, checklists, pocket cards, and chart stickers can help improve HF management.[6] Leveraging the expertise of the interdisciplinary team is central to success. Recognizing the pharmacist's knowledge of pharmacologic properties, trial data and guidelines, and economic feasibility, in addition to their ability to counsel patients extensively can help providers know when to up-titrate the dose and have confidence in what has been demonstrated to be true in clinical trials. Similarly, advanced practice providers are often members of specialized heart failure teams, serving as clinicians and a resource to assist with guideline application, patient counseling, and navigating access issues.

PATIENT FACTORS

Despite strong clinical evidence and patient counseling, socioeconomic factors influence overall patient acceptability, understanding, and accessibility of GDMT. Compounding all the current challenges surrounding the initiation and titration of neurohormonal blockade is the increasing complexity of underlying heart failure management (**Table 2**). Additional therapies continue to gain FDA approval and new pathologic targets have been identified to improve symptoms and/or outcomes for patients with HFrEF, such as the sodium–glucose cotransporter-2 (SGLT2) inhibitors and the guanylyl cyclase stimulators.[22] Intuitively, as the medication regimen gets more complex, adherence declines. Patients can more easily manage simplified regimens with limited therapies and once daily dosing schedules. Additionally, affordability is a constant consideration in light of limited financial resources, not to mention continual efforts by clinical teams to "balance" blood pressure, heart rate, and/or afterload reduction with patient tolerance and avoidance of presyncope and hypotension.

Each patient encounter is an opportunity to escalate GDMT as tolerated, regardless of the type/setting of the encounter. A recent pilot study published by Bhatt and colleagues assessed the possibility of optimizing GDMT through a virtual platform in the setting of a non-HF hospitalization. The team spearheading the initiative, a pharmacist–physician team, provided recommendations on optimization to treating teams. Consequently, findings showed an association in improved GDMT optimization.[23]

As part of shared decision making, patients need comprehensive, repetitive education, and despite best efforts, patients/caregivers remain confused and uncertain about most aspects of the medical regimen. Successful strategies to improve the utilization of GDMT as outlined by well-established guidelines include provider education, patient data collection, and performance feedback. Specific performance improvement activities such as education, reminder systems, profiling, and feedback in real-world clinical practice will identify barriers that limit optimal care delivery.[6] Medication reconciliation at every patient encounter is an established best practice. To promote optimal adherence, routine medication education should reiterate indication, dosing, and potential side effects.

Table 1
Summary of sample literature highlighting percentage of patients with HFrEF at target (100%) doses of GDMT

Name	Literature Category	Percentage of Target Dosing Achieved
IMPROVE-HF[7]	Prospective Observational Study/ Quality Improvement Initiative	ACEI/ARB 37.9%, β-blocker 30.3%, MRA 78.4%[a]
CHAMP-HF[8]	Prospective Observational Study	ACEI/ARB 17.5%, ARNI 14%, β-Blocker 27.5%, MRA 77%
GUIDE-IT[9]	Randomized Multicenter Study	ACEI/ARB 31%, β-blocker 15%, MRA 85%
BIOSTAT-CHF[10]	Multicenter, Multinational, Prospective Observational Study	ACEI/ARB 22%, β-blocker 12%
Diamant et al.[11]	Single-Region Observational Study	ACEI/ARB/ARNI 29%, β-blocker 32%, MRA 4%
QUALIFY[12]	International Prospective Observational Longitudinal Survey	ACEI 27.9%. β-blocker 14.8%, ARB 6.9%, Ivabradine 6.9%
ESC HF Long-term Registry[14]	Multicenter, Prospective Observational Study	ACEI 16.2%, ARB 24%, β-blocker 13.2%, MRA 23.5%
CHECK-HF[15]	Cross-Sectional Dutch Study	RAASI 43.6%, β-blocker 18.9%, MRA 52%

Abbreviations: ACEI, angiotensin-converting enzyme inhibitor; ARB, angiotensin 2 receptor blocker; ARNI, angiotensin receptor neprilysin inhibitor; MRA, mineralocorticoid receptor agonist; β-blocker, beta-blocker; RAASI, renin–angiotensin–aldosterone system inhibitor.
[a] at 24 mo.

Multidisciplinary HF disease management programs are effective in improving quality of care and outcomes in the outpatient setting.[24] However, most patients are not managed by specialized heart failure teams and therefore broad-reaching strategies must be applied across multiple care settings.

Other medical specialties and patient populations face similar challenges. For example, one study in asthma care investigated the impact and experience of using an interactive patient website that offered individual feedback. Patient perspectives were positive, reporting improved communication and interaction with their physicians, suggesting that patients can play a role in overcoming the clinical inertia of providers.[25] Other creative and innovative solutions are needed to overcome this phenomenon and should be considered for further research. Individualized patient care strategies can promote long-term adherence and quality of life. "**Clinics Care Points**" to promote adherence and regimen optimization include:[6,26,27]

- Minimize diuretics to the lowest possible dose to maintain euvolemia
- Avoid the up-titration of neurohormonal blockade if volume depleted or in acute decompensated heart failure (ADHF)
- Space medication dosing to avoid excessive fluctuations in blood pressure or hypotension
- Simplify the dosing regimen when possible (daily dosing vs multiple doses)
- Initiate at low doses and up titrate slowly ("start low, go slow") recognizing there are cumulative benefits of ARNI/BB/MRA/SGLT2i within 30 days of initiation[28]
- Monitor serial laboratories to assess renal function and electrolytes
- Trend biomarkers to assist with clinical decision-making and determine response to therapy (ie, BNP, NTproBNP, troponin)

Table 2
Pathophysiological targets and treatments in HFrEF[22]

Therapy Target	Agent
RAAS inhibition	ACEI, ARB, ARNI, MRA
SNS inhibition	Beta-blockers (ie, Bisoprolol, Carvedilol, Metoprolol Succinate)
SGLT2 inhibition	SGLT2 inhibitors (ie, dapagliflozin and empagliflozin)
Guanylyl cyclase enhancement	Soluble guanylyl cyclase stimulators (ie, vericiguat)
HR/HF hospitalization reduction: Beta-adrenergic receptors Sodium/potassium ATPase pump HCN-gated channel	Beta-blockers Cardiac glycosides (ie, Digoxin) HCN-gated channel inhibitor (ie, Ivabradine)
Congestion: Sodium inhibition in the nephron	Diuretics (Loops, Thiazides)
Vasodilation: Arterioles (afterload) Intracellular cyclic-GMP (preload)	Hydralazine/Nitrates (African Americans, or ACE/ARB/ARNI intolerant)

Abbreviations: RAAS, renin–angiotensin–aldosterone system; SNS, sympathetic nervous system; ACEI, angiotensin-converting enzyme inhibitor; ARB, angiotensin 2 receptor blocker; ARNI, angiotensin receptor neprilysin inhibitor; MRA, mineralocorticoid receptor agonist; SGLT-2, sodium-glucose cotransport-2; HR, heart rate; HF, heart failure; HCN, hyperpolarization-activated cyclic nucleotide; DCT, distal convoluted tubule; GMP, guanosine monophosphate.

- Confirm affordability and access to prescribed medication regimen
- Assess health literacy of every patient and tailor repetitive education and counseling to individual patient needs
- Use "teach back" method to assess recall and understanding—include caregivers in patient education
- Use visual aids and materials to promote further understanding
- Assess all pharmacotherapies on the patient's list for possible drug–drug interactions that can exacerbate negative symptoms. Discontinue/streamline whereby possible

SYSTEM FACTORS

The economic burden of heart failure continues to increase, as the population diagnosed with HF is expected to exceed 8 million by 2030.[29] Heart failure does not occur in a silo. Most patients have multiple comorbidities, thus increasing the complexity and cost of care. Many Medicaid programs also have "limits" on the number of covered prescriptions, thus creating a dilemma for patients who have insufficient financial resources. The American Heart Association (AHA) reports that on average, patients with HF take 6.8 prescription medications per day or approximately 10 doses per 24-h period.[30]

Some of the newer therapies, such as sacubitril/valsartan, dapagliflozin, and vericiguat, are more expensive than long-serving standard therapy, creating a financial burden for many patients and further limiting the utilization of GDMT. Commercial prior authorization programs increase staff workload requirements and further limit patient access to desired therapies. Cost reduction measures include copay assistance programs, as well as price matching between pharmacies. Clinicians must consider the cost-effectiveness of any new therapy to justify the out-of-pocket costs.[22]

Randomized trials have demonstrated the superiority of team-based care in patients with heart failure. These outcomes are generally attributed to greater adherence and up-titration of GDMT.[30–32] One essential skill of HF teams includes treatment prescription, titration, and monitoring, clearly aligned with the scope and expertise of pharmacists.[22,33,34] Many successful transitions of care programs and discharge clinics are either pharmacist and/or Advanced Practice Provider (APP)-driven, which can assist with initiation, titration, and access of GDMT shortly after inpatient discharge.[35] A study conducted by Attar and colleagues comparing GDMT optimization in a pharmacist-led HF clinic versus usual care found that on average after hospital discharge, patient follow-up was within 15 days with a pharmacist versus 31 days with a cardiologist. Additionally, GDMT at target doses was achieved in 59% of patients in the pharmacist group versus 11.4% in the cardiologist group by 3 months.[33]

CONCLUSION

Despite extensive clinical trial experience and clear recommendations from published guidelines, there remains a residual treatment gap in many eligible patients who fail to receive indicated therapies to improve patient outcomes. This is a noted problem across the New York Heart Association (NYHA) spectrum. Earlier referrals to heart failure disease management programs could counteract this inertia and improve adherence to guideline recommendations.[24] Clearly the barriers to optimal medical management are multifactorial and interlinked, creating the "perfect storm" that limits the initiation and up-titration of therapies well-known to improve heart failure outcomes. Multidisciplinary teams that include physicians, APPs, nurses, and pharmacists are best suited to address the many needs of the heart failure population. Keys to success include the following "Clinics Care Points":

- Frequent assessment of volume status and other signs and symptoms of heart failure decompensation
- Evaluation of clinical, social, and financial barriers to achieving GDMT
- Shared decision making that aligns medical therapy with patient values, goals, and preferences[22]
- Incorporation of interdisciplinary team services (eg, pharmacy services) within the practice setting
- Coordination of care between multiple providers to address/limit competing priorities
- Implementation of innovative tools, such as smartphone applications, interactive patient websites, and electronic health record solutions

Data reported in CHAMP-HF and multiple other trials and registries underline the urgency and importance of improving the utilization of GDMT in the heart failure population. It has been estimated that the implementation of GDMT could prevent almost 70,000 deaths per year.[36] We cannot become complacent. These therapies have been proven repeatedly to improve outcomes. This is a far-reaching, complex problem that requires ongoing attention and research. Multidisciplinary teams will play a key role in identifying and implementing effective, innovative strategies, creating a "win-win" for both patients and clinicians.

Perfect Storm.... barriers to GDMT.

DISCLOSURE

S. Dunham and B.T. Davidson do not have any conflicts of interest relative to this work. The authors have not received any funding for this work.

REFERENCES

1. Greene SJ, Adusumalli S, Albert NM, et al. Building a heart failure clinic: a practical Guide from the heart failure Society of America. J Card Fail 2021;27(1):2–19.
2. Benjamin EJ, Muntner P, Alonso A, et al. Heart Disease and Stroke Statistics-2019 Update: a Report From the American Heart Association [published correction appears in Circulation. Circulation 2019;139(10):e56–528, 2020 Jan 14;141(2):e33.
3. O'Connor CM. Guideline-directed medical therapy clinics: a Call to action for the heart failure team. JACC Heart Fail 2019;7(5):442–3.
4. O'Connor PJ, Sperl-Hillen JM, Johnson PE, et al. Clinical inertia and outpatient medical Errors. In: Henriksen K, Battles JB, Marks ES, et al, editors. Advances in patient Safety: from Research to implementation (volume 2: Concepts and methodology). Rockville (MD): Agency for Healthcare Research and Quality (US); 2005.
5. Verhestraeten C, Heggermont WA, Maris M. Clinical inertia in the treatment of heart failure: a major issue to tackle. Heart Fail Rev 2020. https://doi.org/10.1007/s10741-020-09979-z [published online ahead of print, 2020 May 30].
6. Fonarow GC, Albert NM, Curtis AB, et al. Improving evidence-based care for heart failure in outpatient cardiology practices: primary results of the registry to Improve the Use of Evidence-Based Heart Failure Therapies in the Outpatient Setting (IMPROVE HF). Circulation 2010;122:585–96.
7. Gheorghiade M, Albert NM, Curtis AB, et al. Medication dosing in outpatients with heart failure after implementation of a practice-based performance improvement intervention: findings from IMPROVE HF. Congest Heart Fail 2012;18(1):9–17.
8. Greene SJ, Butler J, Albert NM, et al. Medical therapy for heart failure with reduced ejection fraction: the CHAMP-HF registry. J Am Coll Cardiol 2018; 72(4):351–66.
9. Felker GM, Anstrom KJ, Adams KF, et al. Effect of Natriuretic Peptide-Guided therapy on hospitalization or Cardiovascular mortality in high-risk patients with heart failure and reduced ejection fraction: a randomized clinical trial. JAMA 2017;318(8):713–20.
10. Ouwerkerk W, Voors AA, Anker SD, et al. Determinants and clinical outcome of uptitration of ACE-inhibitors and beta-blockers in patients with heart failure: a prospective European study. Eur Heart J 2017;38(24):1883–90.
11. Diamant MJ, Virani SA, MacKenzie WJ, et al. Medical therapy doses at hospital discharge in patients with existing and de novo heart failure. ESC Heart Fail 2019;6(4):774–83.
12. Komajda M, Anker SD, Cowie MR, et al. Physicians' adherence to guideline-recommended medications in heart failure with reduced ejection fraction: data from the QUALIFY global survey. Eur J Heart Fail 2016;18:514–22.
13. Komajda M, Cowie MR, Tavazzi L, et al. Physicians' guideline adherence is associated with better prognosis in outpatients with heart failure with reduced ejection fraction: the QUALIFY international registry. Eur J Heart Fail 2017;19(11):1414–23.
14. Crespo-Leiro MG, Segovia-Cubero J, González-Costello J, et al. Adherence to the ESC heart failure treatment guidelines in Spain: ESC heart failure long-term registry. Rev Esp Cardiol (Engl Ed 2015;68(9):785–93.
15. Brunner-La Rocca HP, Linssen GC, Smeele FJ, et al. Contemporary drug treatment of chronic heart failure with reduced ejection fraction: the CHECK-HF registry. JACC Heart Fail 2019;7(1):13–21.

16. Khan MS, Fonarow GC, Ahmed A, et al. Dose of angiotensin-converting enzyme inhibitors and angiotensin receptor blockers and outcomes in heart failure: a meta-analysis. Circ Heart Fail 2017;10(8):e003956.
17. Calvin JE, Shanbhag S, Avery E, et al. Adherence to evidence-based guidelines for heart failure in physicians and their patients: lessons from the Heart Failure Adherence Retention Trial (HART). Congest Heart Fail 2012;18(2):73–8.
18. Fuat A, Hungin AP, Murphy JJ. Barriers to accurate diagnosis and effective management of heart failure in primary care: qualitative study. BMJ 2003; 326(7382):196.
19. Phillips LS, Branch WT, Cook CB, et al. Clinical inertia. Ann Intern Med 2001; 135(9):825–34.
20. Aujoulat I, Jacquemin P, Rietzschel E, et al. Factors associated with clinical inertia: an integrative review. Adv Med Educ Pract 2014;5:141–7. Published 2014 May 8.
21. Packer M, Metra M. Guideline-directed medical therapy for heart failure does not exist: a non-judgmental framework for describing the level of adherence to evidence-based drug treatments for patients with a reduced ejection fraction. Eur J Heart Fail 2020;22(10):1759–67.
22. Maddox TM, Januzzi JL, Allen LA, et al. 2021 Update to the 2017 ACC Expert consensus decision pathway for optimization of heart failure treatment: Answers to 10 Pivotal issues about heart failure with reduced ejection fraction: a report of the American College of cardiology solution Set Oversight Committee. J Am Coll Cardiol 2021;77(6):772–810.
23. Bhatt AS, Varshney AS, Nekoui M, et al. Virtual optimization of guideline-directed medical therapy in hospitalized patients with heart failure with reduced ejection fraction: the IMPLEMENT-HF pilot study [published online ahead of print, 2021 mar 26]. Eur J Heart Fail 2021. https://doi.org/10.1002/ejhf.2163.
24. McAlister FA, Stewart S, Ferrua S, et al. Multidisciplinary strategies for the management of heart failure patients at high risk for admission: a systematic review of randomized trials. J Am Coll Cardiol 2004;44(4):810–9.
25. Hartmann CW, Sciamanna CN, Blanch DC, et al. A website to improve asthma care by suggesting patient questions for physicians: qualitative analysis of user experiences. J Med Internet Res 2007;9(1):e3.
26. Davidson BT, Allison TL. Improving heart failure patient outcomes utilizing guideline-directed therapy. Nurse Pract 2017;42(7 Suppl 1):2–14.
27. Dunham S, Lee E, Persky AM. The Psychology of following Instructions and its Implications. Am J Pharm Educ 2020;84(8):ajpe7779.
28. Greene SJ, Butler J, Fonarow GC. Simultaneous or rapid sequence initiation of quadruple medical therapy for heart failure—optimizing therapy with the need for speed. JAMA cardiology 2021;6.7:743–4.
29. Benjamin EJ, Virani SS, Callaway CW, et al. Heart Disease and Stroke Statistics-2018 Update: a Report From the American Heart Association [published correction appears in Circulation. Circulation 2018;137(12):e67–492, 2018 Mar 20;137(12):e493.
30. Page RL, Cheng D, Dow TJ, et al. Drugs that may cause or exacerbate heart failure: a scientific statement from the American Heart Association. Circulation 2016; 134:e32–69.
31. Rich MW, Beckham V, Wittenberg C, et al. A multidisciplinary intervention to prevent the readmission of elderly patients with congestive heart failure. N Engl J Med 1995;333(18):1190–5.

32. Phillips CO, Wright SM, Kern DE, et al. Comprehensive discharge planning with postdischarge support for older patients with congestive heart failure: a meta-analysis [published correction appears in JAMA 2004 Sep 1;292(9):1022]. JAMA 2004;291(11):1358–67.

33. Schulz M, Griese-Mammen N, Anker SD, et al. Pharmacy-based interdisciplinary intervention for patients with chronic heart failure: results of the PHARM-CHF randomized controlled trial. Eur J Heart Fail 2019;21(8):1012–21.

34. Koelling TM, Johnson ML, Cody RJ, et al. Discharge education improves clinical outcomes in patients with chronic heart failure. Circulation 2005;111(2):179–85.

35. Attar D, Lekura J, Kalus JS, et al. Impact of A Pharmacist-Led heart failure clinic on guideline-directed medical therapy. J Card Fail 2020;26(10):S129 (suppl).

36. Fonarow GC, Yancy CW, Hernandez AF, et al. Potential impact of optimal. Implementation of evidence-based heart failure therapies on mortality. Am Heart J 2011;161(6):1024–30.

Role of Telemedicine in Improving Guideline-Directed Medical Treatment for Patients with Heart Failure During a Pandemic

Lara S. Hernandez, DNP, APRN, FNP-C

KEYWORDS

- Telehealth • Heart failure • Guideline medications • COVID-19

KEY POINTS

- Telehealth and heart failure
- Heart failure and COVID-19
- Heart failure guidelines
- Adherence to heart failure treatment guidelines

The coronavirus disease 2019 (COVID-19) pandemic has complicated the management of heart failure (HF), which is by itself an intricate disease to treat. Decreased medical contact, reduced social interactions, and lockdowns during this global pandemic are a few of the many factors that have made treating this medically fragile population more complex. In addition, parallels between COVID-19 infection and resulting myocardial injury have been suggested, which may further impair cardiac function and increase exacerbations.[1] Finding innovative strategies to successfully treat patients with HF while keeping them safe from COVID-19 exposure is an unavoidable challenge many providers face while battling this complex virus.

DISCUSSION

Current guideline-directed medical treatment (GDMT) for patients with HF includes the use of Entresto, an angiotensin receptor-neprilysin inhibitor (ARNI), a β-blocker (Metoprolol Succinate, Carvedilol, or Bisoprolol), an aldosterone antagonist (AA), and a sodium-glucose cotransport-2 inhibitor (SGLT-2). This regimen is complex for the

East Jefferson General Hospital Heart Failure Clinic, 4224 Houma Blvd, Suite 500, Metairie, LA 70006, USA
E-mail address: lara.hernandez@lcmchealth.org

Crit Care Nurs Clin N Am 34 (2022) 151–156
https://doi.org/10.1016/j.cnc.2022.02.004
0899-5885/22/© 2022 Elsevier Inc. All rights reserved.

Abbreviations	
COVID-19	coronavirus disease 2019
GDMT	guideline-directed medical treatment
ARNI	Angiotensin receptor-neprilysin inhibitor
B-Blocker	Beta blocker
AA	Aldosterone antagonist
SGLT-2	Sodium-glucose cotransport-2 inhibitor
HF	Heart failure
HFrEF	Heart failure with a reduced ejection fraction
EF	Ejection fraction

patient and provider alike. Patients with HF struggle with polypharmacy and providers battle multiple comorbidities that complicate the initiation and titration of many of the guideline-directed medications. Add in a global pandemic and achieving target or optimal doses of these medications seems like an insurmountable feat.

COVID-19 and Chronic HF

Chronic comorbidities increase the risk of severe COVID-19 and experience a worse prognosis and a mortality rate of over 10%.[2] Viral infections such as coronaviruses and influenza have been shown to exacerbate preexisting HF and increase HF-related hospitalizations. Severe COVID-19 infections necessitate increased cardiac performance and high cardiac output, something that patients with HF are mostly unable to produce. According to Bader and colleagues,[2] established HF is an independent predictor of in-hospital death for COVID-19–infected patients.

Comorbidities

More than half of all patients with HF are diagnosed with 5 or more comorbid conditions, which compound the risk of all-cause and HF hospitalizations. The most common comorbidities found in patients with HF are hypertension (85.6%), ischemic heart disease (72.1%), hyperlipidemia (62.6%), anemia (51.2%), diabetes mellitus (47.1%), arthritis (45.6%), chronic renal insufficiency (CRI; 44.8%), chronic airway diseases (30.9%), and atrial fibrillation (28.8%).[3] CRI is the largest predictor of HF outcome outside left ventricular ejection fraction. Optimal dosing of guideline-directed medications, especially renin-aldosterone-angiotensin blockers, becomes problematic when the glomerular nitration rate is low. Chronic obstructive pulmonary disease (COPD) affects one-third of all patients with HF and predicts mortality. This comorbid condition often goes undiagnosed due to dyspnea, a common finding in patients with HF, being the most frequently reported complaint. There is an underutilization of β-blockers and increased usage of steroids, which increase fluid retention in the COPD population.[3]

Polypharmacy

Owing to the sizable percentage of patients with HF with multiple comorbid conditions, polypharmacy, which is needing to take 5 or more medications daily, is common. Polypharmacy is associated with disability, decreased functional status, and higher incidence of drug-drug interaction effects.[4] The complex medication regimen currently recommended to reduce HF mortality consists of at least 6 medications dosed up to 3 times daily. Combine that with medications used to manage other comorbid conditions, and the result is an overwhelming daily routine that patients struggle to maintain.

Telemedicine and HF

Telemedicine, the practice of delivering health care at a distance using telecommunications technologies, has increased in response to the COVID-19 pandemic. Telemedicine can safely decrease HF hospitalizations, mortality, and risk of exposure to COVID-19.[5] The Heart Failure Society of America released a statement in favor of establishing virtual visits for patients with HF to ensure that the risk of COVID-19 infection is decreased while continuing to provide proper and safe follow-up for this cohort. Bader and colleagues reported that the use of telemedicine produced a decrease in the percentage of no-show visits for hospital follow-up visits 7 days after discharge (51% no-show for in-person vs 34.6% for virtual visits). Limited assessment of clinical volume overload (edema or jugular venous distension) paired with recording of daily weights, vitals, and activity tolerance can also aid in assessing symptoms and guide any medication changes. Telemedicine allows patients with chronic HF to have access to care while decreasing the risk of exposure and further spread of the virus (**Fig. 1**).

Telemedicine and GDMT

A systematic review by Yun and colleagues[5] reported that telemonitoring patients with HF produces a 19% decrease in all-cause mortality but no change in the rate of hospitalization. Medication adherence and early symptom management were the most-reported reasons for the significant reduction in mortality. A randomized controlled trial by Comin-Colet and colleagues[6] demonstrated that HF management using telehealth increased treatment adherence among patients, decreased rehospitalizations, and lowered health-related costs. Blood and colleagues[7] stated that remote monitoring via telehealth with or without video of patients with HFrEF for uptitration of GDMT medications is feasible and cost-effective, given the titration program has specific algorithms for titration and are collaborative between a physician, a pharmacist, and an HF nurse.

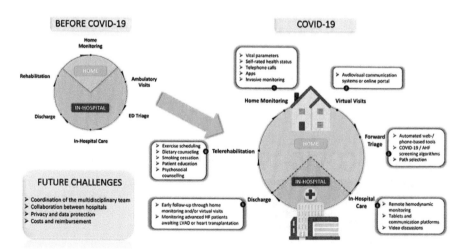

Fig. 1. Telemedicine in patients with heart failure before and during COVID-19. (*From* Tersalvi G, Winterton D, Cioffi GM, Ghidini S, Roberto M, Biasco L, Pedrazzini G, Dauw J, Ameri P and Vicenzi M (2020) Telemedicine in Heart Failure During COVID-19: A Step Into the Future. Front. Cardiovasc. Med. https://www.frontiersin.org/articles/10.3389/fcvm.2020.612818/full. Published December 2020. Accessed 10/01/2021.)

Implementation of Telemedicine During COVID-19

Telehealth is not new to health care providers; it was first used in the 1950s when several hospitals shared images and information via telephone.[8] Before the outbreak of COVID-19, most health systems in the United States had low rates of telehealth use for ambulatory patient care. Many health care facilities have increased telehealth visits from less than 100 per day before the pandemic to more than 1000 visits per day currently (**Fig. 2**). Evidence on the use of telehealth for HF management is sparse and controversial because of the underutilization of telehealth until very recently.[9] Although current findings support the use of telehealth for adults with HF, a meta-analysis by Zhu and colleagues[10] suggests that further research is needed to confirm these results.

Hernandez[11] discovered through a retrospective chart review that telehealth was successful in increasing the number of patients with HFrEF on the appropriate GDMT medications and decreasing HF hospitalizations. The findings also highlighted opportunities for education about the GDMT medications and their appropriate use. The results of this project also provided evidence that it is possible to initiate these medications despite comorbidities. Her[11] review found a 5% increase in patients on appropriate GDMT medications, and this is consistent with the current evidence regarding chronic illness management using telehealth. A systematic review by Kruse and colleagues[12] found that using telehealth for cardiovascular disease management reduced hospital admissions and readmissions but failed to find statistical significance from any of the included articles. Greenhalgh and colleagues[13] found through their systematic review that telehealth was superior in disease-modifying medication titration to higher, more effective doses as compared with standard care.

Telehealth can be used to manage the full spectrum of patients with HF, including those with reduced EF, preserved EF, and across all stages (A-D). The visits can manage new or worsening symptoms of HF, medication titration, hospital discharge follow-up, and new test results. Health care workers represent 20% of COVID-19

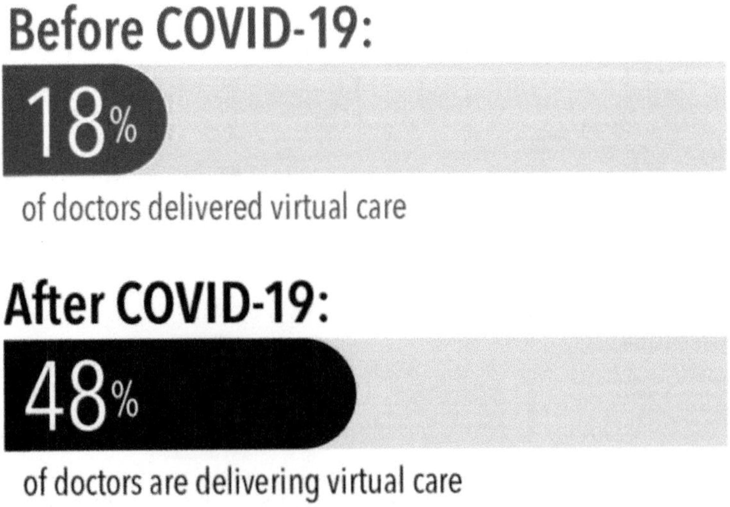

Fig. 2. Rapid adoption in response to COVID-19. (*From* Ed Lee, MD, MPH. How COVID-19 created a telehealth surge. Kaiser Permanente Business. https://business.kaiserpermanente.org/insights/telehealth/covid-19-accelerated-telehealth. Published July 28, 2020. Accessed 10/01/2021.)

cases, and telehealth allows providers who require quarantine but remain well to continue to manage patients.[14] Patients with HF experience many barriers to attending in-person visits, including poor exercise tolerance, difficulty in transporting oxygen, and lack of transportation. Telehealth removes these hurdles, and many believe it will become the norm after the COVID-19 crisis.[14]

SUMMARY

The use of GDMT for improving HFrEF outcomes is well supported by current practice guidelines and evidence. However, recent literature shows that adherence to the guidelines for HFrEF treatment remains low for the provider and patient. Telehealth removes barriers to care for patients with HF and has demonstrated lower hospitalization rates and increased patient satisfaction. Treatment adherence is increased when telehealth is used, and this leads to better success with GDMT titration. Owing to the COVID-19 pandemic, many health care systems quickly implemented telehealth to continue to manage the HF population while reducing potential COVID-19 exposure. GDMT utilization will increase, and hospitalizations will decrease with the use of telehealth despite COVID-19.

CLINICS CARE POINTS

- Telehealth allows providers who require quarantine but remain well to continue to manage patients.[14]
- Patients with HF experience many barriers to attending in-person visits, including poor exercise tolerance, difficulty in transporting oxygen, and lack of transportation, and telehealth removes these hurdles.[14]
- A systematic review by Zhu and colleagues[10] reported that telemonitoring patients with HF produces a 19% decrease in all-cause mortality but no change in the rate of hospitalization
- Telemedicine safely reduces health care use by reducing emergency room visits.[10]
- Telemedicine medication titrations are just as successful as traditional, in-person titrations.[10]

DISCLOSURE

The author has nothing to disclose.

REFERENCES

1. Tersalvi G, Winterton D, Cioffi GM, et al. Telemedicine in heart failure during COVID-19: a step into the future. Front Cardiovasc Med 2020;7:313. https://doi.org/10.3389/fcvm.2020.612818. Accessed September 25, 2021.
2. Bader F, Manla Y, Atallah B, et al. Heart failure and COVID-19. Heart Fail Rev 2021;26:1–10. https://doi.org/10.1007/s10741-020-10008-2. Accessed September 25, 2021.
3. Iyngkaran P, Liew D, Neil C, et al. Moving from heart failure guidelines to clinical practice: gaps contributing to readmissions in patients with multiple comorbidities and older age. Clin Med Insights Cardiol 2018;1–13. https://doi.org/10.1177/1179546818809358. Accessed October, 2021.
4. Bhatt AS, Niteesh CK. Evidence-based prescribing and polypharmacy for patients with heart failure. Ann Intern Med 2021;1–3. https://doi.org/10.7326/M21-1427. Accessed September 25, 2021.

5. Yun JE, Park JE, Park HY, et al. Comparative effectiveness of telemonitoring versus usual care for heart failure: a systematic review and meta-analysis. J Card Fail 2018;24(1):19–28. https://doi.org/10.1016/j.cardfail.2017.09.006. Accessed September 27, 2021.

6. Comín-Colet J, Enjuanes C, Verdú-Rotellar JM, et al. Impact on clinical events and healthcare costs of adding telemedicine to multidisciplinary disease management programmes for heart failure: results of a randomized controlled trial. J Telemed Telecare 2016;22(5):282–95. Accessed September 25, 2021.

7. Blood AJ, Fischer CM, Fera LE, et al. Rationale and design of a navigator-driven remote optimization of guideline-directed medical therapy in patients with heart failure with reduced ejection fraction. Clin Cardiol 2019;43(1):4–13. https://doi.org/10.1002/clc.23291. Accessed September 27, 2021.

8. Teoli D, Aeddula NR. Telemedicine. *NCBI* Bookshelf; 2020. Available at: https://www.ncbi.nlm.nih.gov/books/NBK535343/. Accessed October 1, 2021.

9. Wosik J, Fudim M, Cameron B, et al. Telehealth transformation: COVID-19 and the rise of virtual care. J Am Med Inform Assoc 2020;27(6):957–62. Accessed September 27, 2021.

10. Zhu Y, Gu X, Xu C. Effectiveness of telemedicine systems for adults with heart failure: a meta-analysis of randomized controlled trials. Heart Fail Rev 2020;25:231–43. https://doi.org/10.1007/s10741-019-09801-5. Accessed September 27, 2021.

11. Hernandez L. The impact of telehealth on guideline directed medical treatment for people with heart failure. Lafayette, Louisiana: Diss. University of Louisiana at Lafayette; 2021. Available at: https://www.proquest.com/openview/b26fb45dd140a3b166e0146ab181d3fc/1?pq-origsite=gscholar&cbl=18750&diss=y. Accessed October 1, 2021.

12. Kruse C, Fohn J, Wilson N, et al. Utilization barriers and medical outcomes commensurate with the use of telehealth among older adults: systematic review. JMIR Med Inform 2020;8(8):e20359. Available at: https://doi.org/10.2196/20359. Accessed September 25, 2021.

13. Greenhalgh T, A'Court C, Shaw S. Understanding heart failure; explaining telehealth – a hermeneutic systematic review. BMC Cardiovasc Disord 2017;17:156. https://doi.org/10.1186/s12872-017-0594-2. Accessed September 27, 2021.

14. Gorodeski EZ, Goyal P, Cox ZL, et al. Virtual visits for care of patients with heart failure in the era of COVID-19: a statement from the Heart Failure Society of America. J Card Fail 2020;26(6):448–56. https://doi.org/10.1016/j.cardfail.2020.04.008. Accessed September 27, 2021.

Depression and Heart Failure Assessment, Treatment, and Interventions to Improve Self-Care Behaviors

Linda L. Wick, MSN, APRN, CHFN*

KEYWORDS

- Heart failure • Depression • Screening • Therapy • Self-care

KEY POINTS

- Many heart failure patients have untreated depression.
- Nurses should use evidence-based depression screening tools, such as the PHQ-2 and PHQ-9, to identify patients with possible depression for evaluation by a physician, advanced practice provider, or mental health practitioner.
- Once heart failure patients are diagnosed with depression, nursing opportunities for education include the delayed effect of pharmacologic treatment with SSRI medications as well as the benefits of all therapies for depression.
- Treatment of depression in heart failure patients can improve self-care and thus important patient outcomes, such as morbidity and mortality.

Depression is a major cause of morbidity and mortality in all disease states. One in 5 Americans will suffer a major depressive disorder in their lifetime.[1] The COVID-19 pandemic has exacerbated the mental health crisis and experts expect these numbers to increase. In patients with cardiovascular disease, specifically heart failure, the rates of depression are 20% to 50%, depending on how the severity of depression is measured.[2] Depression and anxiety in heart failure are associated with adverse outcomes, such as decreased adherence to medications and diet, increased hospitalizations or emergency department visits, and even death.[3] In addition to increased morbidity and mortality, the cost of treating heart failure patients with untreated depression is also higher.[4] Heart failure care is currently costing Medicare billions of dollars. The cost of caring for heart failure patients, to Medicare in 2012, was 30.7 billion dollars. This cost is expected to increase to 69.7 billion dollars by 2030.[5] Unfortunately, depression is often untreated in heart failure patients. There are many

Fairview Health Services, American Association of Heart Failure Nurses, 2450 Riverside Ave, Minneapolis, MN, USA
* 929 Portland Avenue, Unit 2510, Minneapolis, MN 55404.
E-mail address: Linda.wick@fairview.org

Crit Care Nurs Clin N Am 34 (2022) 157–164
https://doi.org/10.1016/j.cnc.2022.02.005
0899-5885/22/© 2022 Elsevier Inc. All rights reserved.

reasons for this, and nurses have a unique opportunity to affect the outcomes in this population.

Screening and treating depression and anxiety are part of recommendations in the AHA/ACC/HFSA Guidelines for how to manage heart failure.[6] However, the multispecialty team members caring for heart failure patients are not well trained in how to screen or how to treat depression. As a result, routine screening is often not done, and subsequently, depression in heart failure patients is often not treated.[7]

Another confounding factor in identifying depression in the heart failure population is the overlap of symptoms. Fatigue, loss of appetite, difficulty sleeping, and difficulty concentrating are symptoms that occur in depressed patients without heart failure and in heart failure patients without depression. As a result, it is difficult to tease apart which disease state is causing an exacerbation of symptoms. Heart failure patients and depression patients also share similar pathologic mechanisms. Natriuretic peptides in heart failure are stimulated in areas of the brain regulating blood pressure and fluid control.[8] These in turn affect mood. Inflammatory processes are present in heart failure and result in ventricular remodeling. Depression is also theorized to cause elevated levels of inflammatory markers.[9] Both depression and heart failure are associated with endothelial dysfunction.[10] Finally, both depression and cardiovascular disease are associated with autonomic dysfunction.[11] Low blood pressure affects cognitive function, and it is difficult to ascertain if changes in cognitive function are due to heart failure with low blood pressure or depression. Often they are attributed to heart failure and depression is overlooked. These similar pathologic mechanisms exacerbate both disease states and is another important reason to screen all heart failure patients for depression.

Screening of depression in the heart failure population is an opportunity for nursing. There are many validated depression screening tools available. Examples include the Beck Depression Inventory (BDI); Center for epidemiologic studies depression scale (CESD); Depression Scale (DEPS); Geriatric Depression Scale (GDS); Cornell Scale Screening Hospital Anxiety and Depression Scale (HADS). A simple 2-question depression screening with the Patient Health Questionnaire-2 (PHQ-2) can be easily done in the office or at the bedside, in acute care, and scheduled to be performed at certain intervals. A positive screening on the PHQ-2 (**Fig. 1**) consists of a positive response to one or both questions and indicates that a more comprehensive screening with the 9-question PQ-9 (**Fig. 2**) be completed.[12] This can be done at routine intervals in the clinics, as heart failure patients are seen frequently in the ambulatory setting. The use of electronic medical records provides the opportunity to use technology to automate scheduling of screening tests, track data and provide research opportunities for nursing, and other disciplines. The government implemented Meaningful Use quality metrics in 2017, which linked payments to certain metrics. Depression screening in the ambulatory setting was one such metric, and this did increase depression screening. However, screening without treatment will not change outcomes. A treatment plan for treating depression is needed to change outcomes in the heart failure population. Often heart failure specialists are reluctant to start antidepressants as they are unfamiliar with the nuances of these medications. Or, they will start an antidepressant and then arrange follow-up in the primary care clinic. Primary care providers are much better equipped to deal with depression medication management. However, if the medication is not started promptly, the depression issue often gets lost in the treatment of the patients' other comorbidities. Patients generally do not like having the diagnosis of depression, do not understand the symptoms of depression, or have been raised with a stigma about the diagnosis of depression (or other mental illness) and will not bring it up unless prompted. In addition to medication treatment, patients need mental health therapy. Currently, the United States has a

Patient Health Questionnaire-2 (PHQ-2)

☒ Share

The PHQ-2 inquires about the frequency of depressed mood and anhedonia over the past two weeks. The PHQ-2 includes the first two items of the PHQ-9.

- The purpose of the PHQ-2 is to screen for depression in a "first-step" approach.
- Patients who screen positive should be further evaluated with the PHQ-9 to determine whether they meet criteria for a depressive disorder.

Over the **last 2 weeks**, how often have you been bothered by the following problems?	Not at all	Several days	More than half the days	Nearly every day
1. Little interest or pleasure in doing things	○ 0	○ +1	○ +2	○ +3
2. Feeling down, depressed or hopeless	○ 0	○ +1	○ +2	○ +3

PHQ-2 score obtained by adding score for each question (total points)

Fig. 1. PHQ-2.

shortage of mental health practitioners, and the backlog to get an appointment can be several months.

Men, in particular, are reluctant to discuss depression. Often the symptoms of depression in men present as irritability and anger.[13] These symptoms are often overlooked as society accepts irritability and anger in men much more readily than it does with women. Men in our society have been socialized to suppress emotions except for irritability and anger. Depression in men can also exhibit anxiety.[14] The combination of these behaviors results in the caregivers feeling more anxious and often less willing to participate in the care of the patient. The Gotland Scale for assessing male depression is helpful in recognizing depression in male patients (**Fig. 3**). Building trust with the patient, regardless of their gender, will help the patient share their emotions and open the conversation around mental health. Nurses have a unique opportunity in the acute care setting because of the amount of time spent at the bedside, to develop trust with patients and families and start the conversation.

Nurses have the opportunity and responsibility to discuss the emotional impact of heart failure with the patient and the caregiver. This often opens the door to discuss symptoms of depression with both the patient and the caregiver. Because of the implicit bias in our society around mental health, patients are reluctant to admit any emotional struggles. Having empathic and fact-based conversations with families helps to remove those barriers. Treating depression with evidence-based care is as important as treating heart failure with evidence-based care. When patients and families understand the pathology of depression and the importance of treatment, they are able to reframe their view of mental illness. Treatment plans should include both pharmacology therapy, psychotherapy, and cognitive behavioral therapy (CBT).

There are many pharmaceuticals on the market for depression.[15] There are nuances to each and it is important for the provider prescribing these medications to understand this. Certain medications help with insomnia (often a common symptom), some antidepressants are better in helping with anxiety. They all have side effects that are important to understand (**Box 1**). The provider will choose one that best fits

PATIENT HEALTH QUESTIONNAIRE (PHQ-9)

NAME:_____   DATE:_____

Over the last *2 weeks*, how often have you been
bothered by any of the following problems?
(use "✓" to indicate your answer)

	Not at all	Several days	More than half the days	Nearly every day
1. Little interest or pleasure in doing things	0	1	2	3
2. Feeling down, depressed, or hopeless	0	1	2	3
3. Trouble falling or staying asleep, or sleeping too much	0	1	2	3
4. Feeling tired or having little energy	0	1	2	3
5. Poor appetite or overeating	0	1	2	3
6. Feeling bad about yourself—or that you are a failure or have let yourself or your family down	0	1	2	3
7. Trouble concentrating on things, such as reading the newspaper or watching television	0	1	2	3
8. Moving or speaking so slowly that other people could have noticed. Or the opposite — being so figety or restless that you have been moving around a lot more than usual	0	1	2	3
9. Thoughts that you would be better off dead, or of hurting yourself	0	1	2	3

add columns _____ + _____ + _____

(Healthcare professional: For interpretation of TOTAL,   TOTAL: _____
please refer to accompanying scoring card).

10. If you checked off *any problems*, how *difficult* have these problems made it for you to do your work, take care of things at home, or get along with other people?	Not difficult at all _____
	Somewhat difficult _____
	Very difficult _____
	Extremely difficult _____

Fig. 2. PHQ-9.

the patient's symptoms, the side effect profile of the drug, and should choose an antidepressant that does not interact with other medications. Specific to cardiology patients, serotonin reuptake inhibitors (SSRI) can affect heart rate variability. In some patients, it causes a decreased resting heart rate, and in others an increased resting

The Gotland Male Depression Scale

| Wolfgang Rutz, M.D., Ph.D. | Zoltán Rihmer, M.D., Ph.D. | Arne Dalteg, Ph.D. |
| Psychiatrist, Visby | Psychiatrist, Budapest | Psychologist, Visby |

English version: Per Bech, Lis Raabæk Olsen, Vibeke Nørholm, Psykiatrisk Forskningsenhed, Hillerød

During the past month, have you or others noticed that your behavior has changed, and if so, in which way?

	Not at all	To some extent	Very true	Extremely so
1. Lower stress threshold/more stressed out than usual	☐	☐	☐	☐
2. More aggressive, outward-reacting, difficulties keeping self-control	☐	☐	☐	☐
3. Feeling of being burned out and empty	☐	☐	☐	☐
4. Constant, inexplicable tiredness	☐	☐	☐	☐
5. More irritable, restless and frustrated	☐	☐	☐	☐
6. Difficulty making ordinary everyday decisions	☐	☐	☐	☐
7. Sleep problems: sleeping too much/too little/restlessly, difficulty falling asleep/waking up early	☐	☐	☐	☐
8. In the morning especially, having a feeling of disquiet/anxiety/uneasiness	☐	☐	☐	☐
9. Overconsumption of alcohol and pills in order to achieve a calming and relaxing effect. Being hyperactive or blowing off steam by working hard and restlessly, jogging or other exercises, under- or over-eating	☐	☐	☐	☐
10. Do you feel your behavior has altered in such a way that neither you yourself nor others can recognize you, and that you are difficult to deal with?	☐	☐	☐	☐
11. Have you felt or have others perceived you as being gloomy, negative, or characterized by a state of hopelessness in which everything looks bleak?	☐	☐	☐	☐
12. Have you or others noticed that you have a greater tendency to self-pity, to be complaining or to seem "pathetic"?	☐	☐	☐	☐
13. In your biological family, is there any tendency towards abuse, depression/dejection, suicide attempts or proneness to behaviour involving danger?	☐	☐	☐	☐

Score
0–13: No signs of depression.
13–26: Depression possible. Specific therapy, including psychopharmacological, possibly indicated.
26–39: Clear signs of depression. Specific therapy, including psychopharmacological, clearly indicated.

Fig. 3. Gotland male depression scale.

heart rate. An important evaluation in adding an antidepressant to a cardiac patient's drug regime is to assess their risk of prolongation of QT interval. This prolongation can potentially cause lethal cardiac arrhythmias. Citalopram is the one SSRI that is avoided in patients who are at risk for prolonged QT interval. Paroxetine is the SSRI that is least likely to cause prolongation of the QT interval and can be used instead in this population. It is important that patients understand that these medications do not have an immediate effect. Patients will need to be on antidepressant medication for 4 to 6 weeks before the provider can accurately assess effectiveness. Depending on the patient's response, the provider may increase the dose or need to change the medication all together. This is often frustrating for patients, as they want a quick fix. Reinforcing the importance of giving these medications time to work is something the nurse can influence.

CBT is much more common in the treatment of depression now than it was in the past due to improved research.[16] CBT involves changing one's thinking patterns. Patients are taught to recognize distortions in thinking, and reevaluate their thoughts based on reality, not perception. Patients gain a better understanding of the thoughts and behaviors of others, build skill to deal with difficult situations, and develop a greater sense of accomplishment in one's own ability. CBT also works with patients to help them change behavior patterns. These include facing fears instead of avoiding them, using role-play to prepare for problematic interactions with others, and learning to calm their mind and relax their body. Patients and their therapists work together to develop a therapy plan individualized to the patient.[17]

Other treatment options for depression include exercise, support groups, and improved social support. Cardiac rehabilitation often serves the dual purpose of

---

Box 1
Possible side effects of antidepressant medication

1 Gastrointesinal (nausea, vomiting, GI bleeding)

2 Hepatotoxicity and hypersensitivity reactions (dermatologic and vascular manifestations)

3 Weight gain and metabolic disturbance

4 Cardiovascular (QT interval prolongation, basal heart rate and HRV, hypertension, orthostatic hypotension)

5 Genitourinary (urinary retention, incontinence)

6 Sexual dysfunction

7 Hyponatremia

8 Osteoporosis and fractures

9 Bleeding

10 Central nervous system (seizure threshold, extrapyramidal side effects, serotonin syndrome, headache, stroke)

11 Sweating

12 Sleep disturbances

13 Affective (apathy, switching into hypomania or mania, paradoxic effects)

14 Suicidality

15 Safety in overdose

16 Discontinuation syndromes

17 Ophthalmic (glaucoma, cataract)

18 Hyperprolactinemia

19 Risk during pregnancy and breast feeding

20 Risk of malignancies

---

education, exercise, and socialization.[18] Heart failure support groups are another avenue to discuss depression and heart failure, providing education to a group is less intimidating for patients—and will make them aware they are not alone. It will also raise awareness of the importance of treating depression and how it impacts their heart failure outcomes.

As medicine becomes more complex, the importance of interdisciplinary team care becomes vital in providing the best evidence-based care to patients. Nurses have the unique opportunity to affect the care and outcomes of heart failure patients who also have depression. Nurses are excellent advocates, educators, and assessors. Nurses are also the most trusted professionals, and patients will often open up to nurses about their emotional concerns that they are reluctant to share with others.

In conclusion, nurses who care for heart failure patients need to be aware of the incidence of depression, how to screen heart failure patients for depression, and have a plan on how to get those patients treated that show signs of depression. Our patients' lives depend on it.

DISCLOSURE

The author has nothing to disclose.

REFERENCES

1. Vos T, Abajobir AA, Abate KH, et al. Global regional, and national incidence, prevalence, and year lives with disability for 328 diseases and injuries for 195 countries, 1990-2016; a systematic analysis for the Global Burden of Disease Study 2016. Lancet 2017;390:1211–59.
2. Rutledge T, Reis VA, Link SE. Depression in heart failure: a meta-analytic review of prevalence, intervention effects and association with clinical outcomes. J Am Coll Cardiol 2006;48:1527–37.
3. Celano CM, Villegas AC, Albanese AM, et al. Depression and anxiety in heart failure: a review. Harv Rev Psychiatry 2018;26(4):175–84.
4. Wallenborn J, Angermann CE. Comorbid depression in heart failure. Herz 2014; 38:587–96.
5. Heidenreich PA, Albert NM, Allen LA, et al, American Heart Association Advocacy Coordinating Committee; Council on Arteriosclerosis, Thrombosis and Vascular Biology; Council on Cardiovascular Radiology and Intervention; Council on Clinical Cardiology; Council on Epidemiology and Prevention; Stroke Council. Forecasting the impact of heart failure in the United States: a policy statement from the american heart association. Circ Heart Fail 2013;6:606–19.
6. 2017 ACC/AHA/HFSA Focused Update of the 2013 ACCF/AHA Guideline for the Management of Heart Failure: A Report of the American College of Cardiology/ American Heart Association Task Force on Clinical Practice Guidelines and the Heart Failure Society of America
7. Huffman JC, Smith FA, Blais MA, et al. Recognition and treatment of depression and anxiety in patients with acute myocardial infarction. Am J Cardiol 2006;98: 319–24.
8. Hu K, Gaudron P, Bahner U, et al. Changes of atrial natriuretic peptide in brain areas of rats with chronic myocardial infarction. Am J Physiol 1996;270:H312–6.
9. Westman PC, Lipinski MJ, Luger D, et al. Inflammation as a Driver of adverse left ventricular remodeling after acute myocardial infarction. J Am Coll Cardiol 2016; 67:20150–60.
10. Kop WJ, Kuhl EA, Barasch E, et al. Association between depressive symptoms and fibrosis markers: the Cardiovascular Health Study. Brain Behav Immun 2010;24:229–35.
11. Fischer D, Rossa S, Landmesser U, et al. Endothelial dysfunction in patients with chronic heart failure is independently associated with increased incidence of hospitalization cardiac transplantation, or death. Eur Heart J 2005;26:65–9, jarni Sigurdsson, Sigurdur Pall Palsson, Olafur Aevarsson, Maria Olafsdottir, Magnus Johannsson.
12. Validity of gotland male depression scale for male depression in a community study: the Sudurnesjamenn study. J Affect Disord 2015;173:81–9. https://doi.org/10.1016/j.jad.2014.10.065. ISS 0165-0327.
13. Carvalho A F, Sharma MS, Brunoni A R, et al. The safety, tolerability and risks associated with the use of newer generation antidepressant drugs: a critical review of the literature. Psychother Psychosom 2016;85:270–88.
14. Dhar AK, Barton DA. Depression and the link with cardiovascaular disease. Front Psychiatry 2016;7:33.
15. National Institute of Mental Health. Available at: http://www.nimh.nih.gov/.

16. Freedland DI, Carney RM, Rich MW, et al. Cognitive behavior therapy for depression and self-care in heart failure patients; a randomized clinical trial. JAMA Intern Med 2015;175:1773–82.

17. David D, Cristea I, Hofmann SG. Why cognitive behavioral therapy is the current gold standard of psychotherapy. Front Psychiatry 2018;9(4). https://doi.org/10.3389/fpsyt.2018.00004.

18. Savage PD, Sanderson BK, Brown TM, et al. Clinical research in cardiac rehabilitation and secondary prevention: looking back and moving forward. J Cardiopulm Rehabil Prev 2011;31(6):333–41.

Treating Sepsis in Patients with Heart Failure

Fiona Winterbottom, DNP, MSN, APRN, ACNS-BC, ACHPN, CCRN

KEYWORDS

- Sepsis • Morbidity • Mortality • Mean arterial pressure • Heart failure

KEY POINTS

- Sepsis is a life-threatening syndrome.
- Early detection and intervention can sreduce sepsis mortality.
- A personalized approach may be beneficial for patients with complex comorbidities.

Sepsis is defined as life-threatening organ dysfunction caused by a dysregulated host response to infection.[1] Morbidity and mortality from sepsis are estimated to affect millions of people annually and it is a significant global public health concern.[1,2] This article discuss treatments recommendations for patients with sepsis and septic shock including those with heart failure.

BACKGROUND

In 2001, a landmark paper was published that described early goal-directed therapy (EGDT) for patients with severe sepsis and septic shock.[3] EGDT was a bundle of interventions that included targets of mean arterial pressure (MAP) greater than 65 mm Hg, central venous pressure (CVP) 8–12 mm Hg, and central venous oxygenation saturation (ScvO2) greater than 70%.[3] The study demonstrated that patients who received EGDT for severe sepsis and septic shock within 6 hours of emergency room presentation had decreased mortality with rates in the standard therapy group of 46.5% and 30.5% in the EGDT group.[3] Since then, several studies have tried to replicate the EGDT study with varying results.[4] Investigators from 3 large sepsis trials, ARISE, ProCESS, and ProMISe, published a systematic review and meta-analysis in an effort to compare reductions in mortality between EGDT and other resuscitation strategies for emergency department (ED) patients presenting with septic shock.[4] The review from 2017 concluded that EGDT was not superior to standard therapy for patients with ED with septic shock but was associated with an increased in use of intensive care unit (ICU) resources.[4] The mortality in the standard therapy group was 22.4% and 23.2% in the EGDT group.[4] The Surviving Sepsis Campaign guidelines

Pulmonary Critical Care, Ochsner Medical Center, New Orleans, LA 70121, USA
E-mail address: fwinterbottom@ochsner.org

Crit Care Nurs Clin N Am 34 (2022) 165–172
https://doi.org/10.1016/j.cnc.2022.02.006
0899-5885/22/© 2022 Elsevier Inc. All rights reserved.

ccnursing.theclinics.com

recommended EGDT from 2004 leading to changes in care practices for patients with severe sepsis and septic shock and possibly leading to a global decrease in mortality from sepsis.[4] In 2016, EGDT was removed from the Surviving Sepsis Campaign guidelines based on the aforementioned sepsis trials.[5] It is important to mention that Centers for Medicare & Medicaid Services' Severe Sepsis and Septic Shock Early Management Bundle (SEP-1) measure was established as a national priority in 2015.[5] While most groups agree on the importance of improving sepsis management and outcomes, there remains debate about standardized regulatory versus guideline-based care interventions.[5] Most of the debate comes down to the nuances of clinician decision-making and individualized patient care.[5] Recommendations for initial resuscitation for those with septic shock includes administration of 30 mLs/kg of balanced crystalloid.[1] There is concern by some clinicians that high doses of volume to patients with heart failure may result in increased mortality.[6,7] The following sections will discuss the care of patients with sepsis and septic shock in the acute care setting.

Screening and Identification

Early identification of sepsis through screening is one of the most effective ways to prevent further deterioration to septic shock. Over the years recommendations have changed as the science around sepsis has evolved. Initial sepsis guidelines included infection, at least 2 systemic inflammatory response syndrome (SIRS) criteria, and new organ dysfunction. Additionally, septic shock included the sepsis criteria plus refractory hypotension of less than a systolic blood pressure of 90 mm Hg or lactate greater than 4. Newer criteria include suspected infection, plus organ dysfunction, and an increase in the SOFA score of ≥ 2 points. See **Box 1** and **Table 1**.

The 2021 international guidelines for the management of sepsis and septic shock issue a strong recommendation for using a performance improvement program that includes sepsis screening and standard operating procedures for treatment.[5] Several innovative multiparameter screens and clinic decision support tools such as the National Early Warning Score (NEWS) and the Modified Early Warning Score (MEWS) are available and being further developed to help clinicians with early identification of sepsis.[1] See **Fig. 1**.

Once integrated into sepsis performance improvement programs and clinical workflows have the power to greatly influence clinical practice and outcomes.[1] Once identified, patient need to receive the appropriate treatment to prevent clinical

---

Box 1
Sepsis definition

Sepsis is life threatening organ dysfunction caused by a dysregulated host response to infection.

- Sepsis clinical criteria:
  - Suspected infection + Organ Dysfunction
  - Organ dysfunction defined as an increase of 2 points or more in the Sequential Organ Failure Assessment (SOFA) score

Septic shock is a subset of sepsis in which underlying circulatory and cellular/metabolic abnormalities are profound enough to substantially increase morality

- Septic shock clinical criteria:
  - Suspected infection + Organ dysfunction and both:
  - Persistent hypotension requiring vasopressors to maintain MAP greater than or equal to 65 mm Hg despite adequate volume resuscitation
  - Lactate greater than or equal to 2 mmol/L

Table 1
Sepsis definitions

Sepsis is defined as at least two of the following signs and symptoms (SIRS) that are both present and new to the patient and suspicion of new infection:

- Hyperthermia >38.3°C or Hypothermia <36°C
- Tachycardia >90 bpm
- Leukocytosis (>12,000 μL-1) or Leukopenia (<4000 μL-1) or >10% bands.

- Acutely Altered Mental Status
- Tachypnea >20 bpm
- Hyperglycemia(>120 mg/dL) in the absence of diabetes

Severe sepsis includes SIRS and at least one of the following signs of hypoperfusion or organ dysfunction that is new and not explained by other known etiology of organ dysfunction:

- Hypotension (<90/60 or MAP <65)
- Areas of mottled skin or capillary refill ≥3 s
- Disseminated intravascular coagulation (DIC)
- Acute renal failure or urine output <0.5 mL/kg/h for at least 2 h
- Cardiac dysfunction

- Lacate >2
- Creatinine >2.0 mg/dL
- Platelet count <100,000
- Hepatic dysfunction as evidenced by Bilirubin >2 or INR >1.5
- Acute lung injury or ARDS

New septic shock is defined as severe sepsis associated with refractory hypotension(BP <90/60) despite adequate fluid resuscitation and/or a serum lactate level ≥4.0 mmol/L

deterioration. This can also be tracked through models that include predictive modeling, artificial intelligence, and clinical decision support.[5]

Interventions and Initial Resuscitation

Initial interventions for patients with suspected sepsis have been placed in care bundles and include measurement of lactate, blood cultures before antibiotics, broad-spectrum antibiotics, fluid resuscitation, and vasopressors.[8] The goal is to have all

Automated Early Warning Scores

	3	2	1	0	1	2	3
RR/min		<8		9–14	15–20	21-29	>30
HR/min		<40	40–50	51–100	91-110	111-129	>130
SBP	<70	71–80	81–100	101-199		>200	
AVPU				Alert	Reacts to Voice	Reacts to Pain	Unresponsive
Temperature (F)		<95	95.1–96.8	96.9–100.4	100.5–101.3	101.4	

Fig. 1. Example of the criteria behind and screenshot of an automated Early Warning Scoring System.

Types of Shock

		Pre-load	Pump Fn	After-load	Perfusion
		PCWP JVP	CO	SVR	O2 Sat
Hypovolemic	- Intravascular vol loss - hemorrhagic - fluid loss	↓	↓	↑	↓
Cardiogenic	- Arrhythmia - AMI, valve failure - cardiomyopathy - pericarditis/PE	↑	↓	↑	↓
Distributive	Vasodilatory-↓↓ SVR -septic shock/SIRS/TSS - Anaphylaxis - neurogenic shock - Drug/toxin - Addisonian crisis	↓/-	↑	↓	-/↑
Obstructive	- Tension PTX - Tamponade - PE	↑	↓	-/↑	-/↓

Fig. 2. Types of shock.

interventions completed within 3 to 6 hours of recognition, but preferably as soon as possible. For those with septic shock, the goal is to administer antibiotics within 1 hour of recognition.[8] Drawing cultures before antibiotic administration increase the yield of the culture and allows for de-escalation once the offending bacteria is isolated. This aligns with good antibiotic stewardship practices. Broad-spectrum antibiotics given in a timely manner can prevent sepsis from worsening to septic shock.

Shock can be described as life-threatening circulatory failure that leads to inadequate cellular oxygen utilization.[9] See **Fig. 2**.

Septic shock is the most common type of shock followed by cardiogenic and hypovolemic shock. Hemodynamics and interventions vary for different types of shock and so it is important to try to differentiate which type of shock state the patient is in.[9]

Initial fluid resuscitation for patients with sepsis-induced hypoperfusion or septic shock is 30 mLs of balanced crystalloid that should be given within the first 3 hours of resuscitation. This amount of fluid is often questioned in certain populations of patients, particularly those with heart failure and end-stage renal disease. Some studies show that patients who did not receive this amount of fluid had increased odds of in-hospital mortality, delayed resolution of hypotension, and increased ICU, regardless of comorbidities.[1]

Several studies report that static measures such as blood pressure or CVP are commonly used to make fluid decisions.[9] The 2021 guidelines suggest using dynamic measures over physical examination or static parameters to guide fluid resuscitation.[1] Physiologic indicators of fluid responsiveness provide a mechanism for targeted resuscitation. Dynamic measures include passive leg raise (PLR) with cardiac output (CO) assessment, fluid challenges with stroke volume (SV), systolic pressure or pulse pressure, and increases of SV with changes in intrathoracic pressure. A 10% increase in SV means that the patient is responsive to fluid and additional fluid should be administered. If there is no change in SV, then vasopressors should be initiated as additional fluid will be unlikely to be beneficial and may be harmful. One systematic review and meta-analysis found that using dynamic assessment to guide fluid therapy was associated with reduced mortality, ICU length of stay, and duration of mechanical ventilation.[1]

Because there is a concern for volume overload and reduced contractility, dynamic assessment measures seem to make sense in preventing over resuscitation. There is some thought that contractility or cardiomyopathy can occur from sepsis in which case Dobutamine may be a consideration.

Protocols and algorithms

There is an ongoing discussion about the best approach to guide resuscitation in groups with multiple comorbidities, including those with heart failure. Standardized, targeted protocols that can be customized to an individual's fluid responsive state may prevent over resuscitation. Examples of this type of algorithm can be found that provide a structured and measurable approach to volume resuscitation in patients with heart failure[9] Initial considerations should be a target at resolving hypotension and shock.[10]

A recent study evaluated fluid responsiveness in hypotension and shock with the primary goal of determining if SV-guided dynamic assessment could guide the amount of IV fluid administered to patients with septic shock.[11] Clinical interventions in the study were guided by a simple algorithm for administering vasopressors or fluid based on a change in SV of less than or more than 10% respectively.[11] The study found that patients in the intervention arm whereby fluid responsiveness was measured, had a lower fluid balance at 72 hours or discharge, required less renal replacement therapy, or mechanical ventilation.[11] These results seem to indicate that a protocolized approach to fluid therapy dosing and assessment of response is an important factor to consider in initial resuscitation.[11]

The overall strategy for patient who is identified as septic follows a simple algorithm that includes treating infection with antibiotics and source control and stabilizing hemodynamics with fluids and vasopressors. See **Figs. 3** and **4**.

Additional Therapies for Sepsis Management

Other sepsis management therapies outlined in the 2021 guidelines include suggestions for ventilation, steroids, restrictive transfusion strategies, veno-thromboembolism

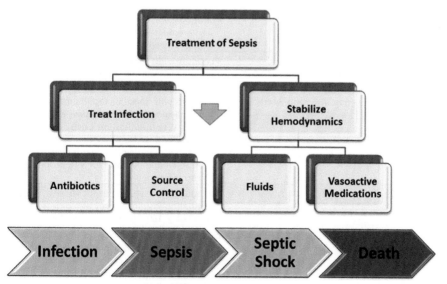

Fig. 3. Outline of sepsis management strategies.

The Four Pillars of Sepsis

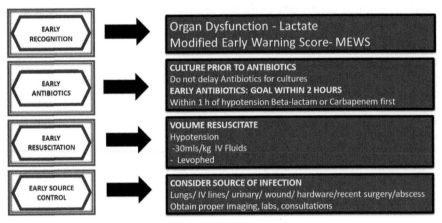

Fig. 4. Sepsis managment Fundamentals.

Table 2
Additional sepsis management therapies

Therapy	Recommendation
Ventilation	Suggest the use of high flow nasal oxygen over non-invasive ventilation
Acute Respiratory Distress Syndrome(ARDS)	Recommend low tidal volume ventilation strategy (6 mL/kg),over a high tidal volume strategy(>10 mL/kg)
Steroids	For adults with septic shock and an ongoing requirement for vasopressor therapy using IV corticosteroids is suggested
Restrictive transfusion strategies	For adults with sepsis and septic shock, a restrictive(over liberal)transfusion strategy is recommended
Venous-thromboembolism prophylaxis	For adults with sepsis or septic shock pharmacologic VTE prophylaxis is suggested unless a contraindication exists For adults with sepsis or septic shock, using low molecular weight heparin over unfractionated heparin for VTE prophylaxis is recommended
Glucose control	For adults with sepsis or septic shock, intitiating insulin therapy at a glucose level of $\geq$ 180 mg/dL (10 mmol/L) is recommended
Long-term outcomes	For adults with sepsis or septic shock, discussing goals of care and prognosis with patients and families over no such discussion is recommended

prophylaxis, glucose levels, and long-term outcomes. This is important to make sure clinical interventions align with patient preferences and values.[1] See **Table 2**.

DISCUSSION

Recommended sepsis management includes volume resuscitation and vasopressor administration for septic shock. Some studies have found that there is no difference in mortality with the delivery of 30 mLs/kg of fluid in septic patients with heart failure.[12,13] Others recommend that protocolized and individualized management may decrease mortality, reduce the length of stay, and improve ventilator outcomes.[12,14] These conflicting discussions cause confusion and can result in patients with comorbidities such as heart failure and end-stage renal disease receive less resuscitation than the guidelines recommend.[6,15] Finally, early low-dose vasopressors may improve clinical outcomes.[16]

SUMMARY

Sepsis guidelines and performance improvement programs have improved mortality from sepsis; however, much research remains to be done to bridge knowledge and practice gaps in the use of technology and nursing care.

CLINICS CARE POINTS

- Guidelines provide a standard for sepsis management
- Protocols can guide care process and practice
- Expert assessment can provide individualized interventions
- Technology can support clinical decision-making

DISCLOSURE

The author has nothing to disclose.

REFERENCES

1. Evans L, Rhodes A, Alhazzani W, et al. Surviving sepsis campaign: international guidelines for management of sepsis and septic shock 2021. Intensive Care Med 2021;47(11):1181–247. https://doi.org/10.1007/s00134-021-06506-y.
2. Rhee C, Dantes R, Epstein L, et al. Incidence and trends of sepsis in US hospitals using clinical vs claims data, 2009–2014. JAMA 2017;318(13):1241–9.
3. Rivers E, Nguyen B, Havstad S, et al. Early goal-directed therapy in the treatment of severe sepsis and septic shock. N Engl J Med 2001;345(19):1368–77.
4. Angus DC, Barnato AE, Bell D, et al. A systematic review and meta-analysis of early goal-directed therapy for septic shock: the ARISE, ProCESS and ProMISe Investigators. Intensive Care Med 2015;41(9):1549–60.
5. Wong A, Otles E, Donnelly JP, et al. External validation of a widely implemented proprietary sepsis prediction model in hospitalized patients. JAMA Intern Med 2021; 181(8):1065–70.
6. Boccio E, Haimovich A, Jacob V, et al. Sepsis fluid metric compliance and its impact on outcomes of patients with congestive heart failure, end-stage renal disease or obesity. J Emerg Med 2021;61(5):466–80.

7. Arfaras-Melainis A, Polyzogopoulou E, Triposkiadis F, et al. Heart failure and sepsis: practical recommendations for the optimal management. Heart Fail Rev 2020;25(2):183–94.

8. Rhee C, Chiotos K, Cosgrove SE, et al. Infectious diseases society of America position paper: recommended revisions to the national severe sepsis and septic shock early management bundle (SEP-1) sepsis quality measure. Clin Infect Dis 2021;72(4):541–52.

9. Kupchik N. Principles of resuscitation. Crit Care Nurs Clin North Am 2021;33(3): 225–44.

10. Ladzinski AT, Thind GS, Siuba MT. Rational fluid resuscitation in sepsis for the hospitalist: a narrative review. InMayo clinic proceedings. Elsevier; 2021.

11. Douglas IS, Alapat PM, Corl KA, et al. Fluid response evaluation in sepsis hypotension and shock: a randomized clinical trial. Chest 2020;158(4):1431–45.

12. Khan RA, Khan NA, Bauer SR, et al. Association between volume of fluid resuscitation and intubation in high-risk patients with sepsis, heart failure, end-stage renal disease, and cirrhosis. Chest 2020;157(2):286–92.

13. Payne WN, II AT, Broce M, et al. An evaluation of the use of aggressive fluid resuscitation in the early treatment of sepsis patients. Cureus 2021;13(2).

14. Taenzer AH, Patel SJ, Allen TL, et al. Improvement in mortality with early fluid bolus in sepsis patients with a history of congestive heart failure. Mayo Clinic Proc Innov Qual Outcomes 2020;4(5):537–41.

15. Jones TW, Smith SE, Van Tuyl JS, et al. Sepsis with preexisting heart failure: management of confounding clinical features. J Intensive Care Med 2021;36(9): 989–1012.

16. Barlow B, Bissell BD. Evaluation of evidence, pharmacology, and interplay of fluid resuscitation and vasoactive therapy in sepsis and septic shock. Shock 2021; 56(4):484–92.

Educating Bachelor of Science in Nursing Students in Leadership Strategies Needed for Care Management and Disease Management for the Heart Failure Patient Population

Jennifer M. Manning, DNS, ACNS-BC, CNE*,
Pam Mattio, BSN, RN, CEN, CPHQ

KEYWORDS

- BSN students • Leadership • Care management • Disease management
- Heart failure

KEY POINTS

- During BSN program education, student nurses are introduced to topics such as heart failure patient care across health care settings, health promotion, safety and quality, technology, and leadership in the health care system as it relates to cardiovascular patients.
- There are various strategies in ensuring BSN students are prepared for providing HF patient care in care management.
- Leadership strategies are included in BSN training to ensure they are prepared for the care management and disease management needs of this population.

INTRODUCTION AND BACKGROUND

The Bachelor of Science in Nursing (BSN) is an undergraduate level degree for registered nurses (RNs).[1-3] During BSN program education, student nurses are introduced to topics such as patient care across health care settings, health promotion, safety and quality, technology, and leadership in the health care system. One area of emphasis is in cardiovascular patient care whereby BSN students develop leadership skills needed for care and disease management for patients with HF.[4]

Nursing schools use various educational strategies to deliver a large amount of educational content to BSN students. Educational delivery methods include didactic

Louisiana State University, Health New Orleans School of Nursing, LCMC Health East Jefferson General Hospital, 4200 Houma Blvd, Metairie, LA 70006, USA
* Corresponding author. 1900 Gravier St, New Orleans, LA 70112.
E-mail address: jmanni@lsuhsc.edu

Crit Care Nurs Clin N Am 34 (2022) 173–180
https://doi.org/10.1016/j.cnc.2022.02.007
0899-5885/22/© 2022 Elsevier Inc. All rights reserved.

ccnursing.theclinics.com

instruction in classroom settings, hands-on education in laboratory and simulation settings, and hands-on clinical training with patients in health care settings. Embedded in these educational methods are skill development for leading in health care settings. The 3 educational methods are needed to ensure BSN students are prepared to provide comprehensive care to a wide variety of patients, such as those with HF.

HF is a chronic disease that requires long-term patient care management. The care of the HF patient is multifaceted. It includes recommendations for regular exercise, smoking cessation, control of hypertension and hyperlipidemia, abstaining from alcohol and recreational drug use, and adherence to medication regimen.[5] The primary patient goal is to slow disease progression, reduce cardiac workload, control fluid retention, and improve cardiac function. BSN graduates need leadership skills to ensure care management and disease management is comprehensive.

The complexity of heart failure patient care

The most common heart disease is coronary artery disease (CAD), whereby there are narrowed arteries and decreased blood flow to the heart, which can result in myocardial infarction (MI). CAD and hypertension gradually leave the heart too weak or stiff to fill and pump blood properly over time. HF contributes to more than 690,000 deaths per year, with sudden death occurring at a rate of six times the general population (CDC, 2021) **(Fig. 1)**. Of the 6 million Americans living with HF, many patients experience a wide variety of physical and emotional symptoms such as edema, fatigue, dyspnea, loss of sleep, depression, and chest pain.[5]

HF is the most common cause of hospital admissions in patients more than 65 and unplanned readmissions in 30 days (Glenn, 2019). The cost of HF continues to rise with an estimated cost of approximately 40 billion per year.[6] The complexity in coordinating care for patients with HF requires adequate discharge planning, consistent medication reconciliation, and effective patient education. Additionally, during transitions in care, patients with HF move from one setting to another, which must be coordinated seamlessly with the support of the health care team. Leadership skills are required to ensure care is delivered most efficiently and effectively.

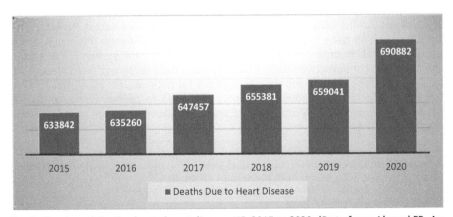

Fig. 1. Number of deaths due to heart disease, US, 2015 to 2020. (*Data from*: Ahmad FB, Anderson RN. The Leading Causes of Death in the US for 2020. JAMA. 2021;325(18):1829 to 1830. https://doi.org/10.1001/jama.2021.5469.)

Strategies for leadership development in Bachelor of Science in Nursing nursing education

Nursing programs use a systematic approach to educating BSN students. Pat Benner, a nursing theorist, developed the *Novice to Expert Theory* which describes an approach for training BSN students whereby the student transitions in skills and competency from a novice to an expert[2] (**Fig. 2**). Strategies to transition students from novice to expert over the course of the BSN program include didactic education, case studies, role play, and simulation.[4] Leadership development outcomes are embedded across the BSN curriculum.[7,8]

Educating BSN students includes a stepwise building as students' progress through the curriculum, transitioning from novice to expert (see **Fig. 2**).[2] In the first year of training, novice students begin with health sciences education related to cardiovascular anatomy, physiology, pathophysiology, and pharmacology. Education is initially provided, which includes normal heart function, types of HF, symptoms of HF, diagnosis, complications, and treatment. Providing evidence-based resources for students in an ever-changing health care field is a crucial step. Exposing students to the best evidence available in cardiovascular patient care such as the American College of Cardiology, American Heart Association, Journal of the American Heart Association, American Journal of Cardiology, National Heart, Lung, and Blood Institute, and the Centers for Disease Control.

As students transition to advanced beginners, they are introduced to chronic case scenarios and patient care settings. Leadership development begins here whereby students learn to provide nursing care, delegate care to unlicensed professionals (ULP), and participate as a member of the interdisciplinary health care team. Considerations for self-care, patient education, transitional care considerations, health literacy, and patient-centered care attitudes should be taught and evaluated for student competency. Students' progress to the competence phase as they are exposed to more acute care areas. They conclude their BSN training by reaching proficiency and possibly expertise in their final year of the program, whereby they take on most of the patient care with direct oversight by a faculty or preceptor.

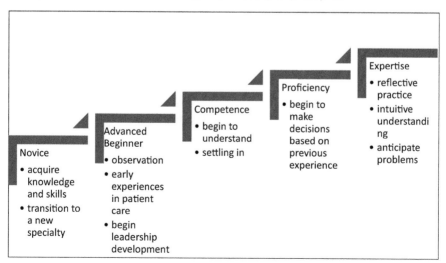

Fig. 2. Application of Benner's novice to expert theory in BSN students. (*From* Transitioning Novice Nurses to Expert Nurses in Progressive Telemetry Care" (2016). Nursing Theses and Capstone Projects. 245. https://digitalcommons.gardner-webb.edu/nursing_etd/245.)

Heart failure care management

Care management refers to a comprehensive, multidisciplinary approach to help care for patients with complex diseases such as HF. There are various strategies in ensuring BSN students are prepared for providing HF patient care in care management. Care management includes several vital areas: face-to-face patient care management, telephone care management, self-management, self-monitoring, and decision support. When care management is provided in these areas, improved outcomes in quality of life, mortality, self-reported health, and self-efficacy are noted[9,10].

BSN Students are introduced to evidence-based strategies to enhance the success of patients with HF after discharge. Such strategies may include education about self-care at home and what action to take when a problem is recognized. The use of teach-back strategies is essential for assessing patient understanding of key concepts and enhancing education strategies when needed. Depression screening should be conducted in all settings to identify and treat this potential barrier to effective self-care. Follow-up phone calls within a few days after hospitalization and an appointment within 1 week with a provider who is focused on the patient's volume status, medication reconciliation, renal function, and other issues are essential. Management of comorbidities are also critical to HF care, and BSN students are made aware of the influence of control of COPD, diabetes, chronic kidney disease, and assessment for and treatment of obstructive sleep apnea have on the success of patients with HF in the hospital and community settings[11–13]

Topics taught to students learning about patients with HF include the 3 "Ps" of holistic cardiovascular patient care: pathophysiology, pharmacology, and physical assessment (**Fig. 3**). Cardiovascular pathophysiology includes topics such as cardiac function, alterations in cardiac function, HF and dysrhythmias, and shock. Cardiovascular pharmacology topics include topics such as cardiac glycosides, antianginals, antidysrhythmics, diuretics, antihypertensives, anticoagulants, antiplatelets, thrombolytics, antihyperlipidemics, and medications to improve peripheral blood flow. Additional guideline-directed medications for patients with HF are included, such as renin–angiotensin–aldosterone inhibitors, beta-blockers, hydralazine, and nitrate combination therapy, and sodium–glucose cotransporter-2 (SGLT2) inhibitors to decrease morbidity and mortality. Cardiovascular physical assessment topics include cardiovascular structure and function, cultural considerations, older adult

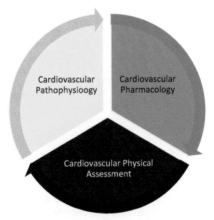

Fig. 3. The 3 "Ps" of holistic cardiovascular patient care.

considerations, assessment of risk factors, screening techniques, comprehensive physical assessment techniques, and critical thinking with laboratory and diagnostic testing.[4]

The best strategies for teaching leadership skills to BSN students include engaging education techniques such as case studies and active learning strategies. The goal is to promote and sustain learning in both academic and clinical settings.[14] Although there is a lack of experimental studies evaluating the effectiveness of education strategies in BSN students, there is a significant number of descriptive, single group

Table 1 **HF case study considerations**	
Case Study Considerations	**Description**
Typical Case Study Components	• Describe the problem • Include supporting data ranging from narrative information about the patient (past medical history, diagnosis, and so forth), laboratory and diagnostic results, patient or caregiver statements, images, video or audio • Include a question or problem to be solved • Leadership Consideration: Describe the leader's role in addressing this problem
Approaches	• Include questions to promote problem-solving • Require decision making in complex situations • Require the student to address ambiguities • Leadership Consideration: Describe how the leader can approach solving this complex problem. Require the student to describe case-based leadership approaches
In the classroom	• Present the case study for analysis • Provide enough information for students to figure out solutions • Identify how solutions can be applied in similar situations (compare) • Identify how solutions are different across various situations (contrast) • Leadership Consideration: Identify leadership strengths and weaknesses
Questions to ask in the case	• What is the patient care issue? • What is the patient care goal? • What is the context of the problem? • What are the key facts for consideration? • What are alternatives available? • What is recommended and why? • Leadership Consideration: How can the leader ensure a building of a wellness culture to ensure maximum return on investment (ROI) in this case?
Individual Assignments	• Provide accompanying reading assignments to introduce or explain the concept • The more complex the topic, the more reading assignments should be assigned • Leadership Consideration: Ensure a leadership question is included based on one of the following topic areas: leadership development, leading high performing teams, leading organizational change, financial considerations for leaders, promoting innovation, identifying opportunities, incorporating evidence-based practice, legal considerations, addressing emerging trends, and incorporating patient-centered innovation. Provide reading assignments on leadership styles and behaviors

studies which can be used to support strategies in the academic learning environment.[7]

The complexity of the care management field lends itself to learning strategies that approach comprehensive patient care, such as with a case study in didactic, simulation, and practicum settings. The advantage in using a case study is students learn through the use of an example rather than learning through principles in general patient care. Case studies can be used in several ways to educate students in the care of complex patients such as those with HF. Leadership techniques can be easily incorporated to direct students to consider not only the care of the patient but the role of the leader in assuring optimal outcomes **(Table 1)**.

Leadership

Leadership development in cardiovascular health requires development through systematic training and mentoring. Achievement of defined skills can be achieved through clear goal identification, team player, problem-solving approach, determination and grit, methodological and practical approaches, rewards, effective communication, and vision.[15]

According to the American Nurses Credentialing Center (ANCC), the transformational leadership style has been identified as the style whereby leaders can organize staff around a collective purpose and drive the organization to realize goals **(Fig. 4)**.[15] Five factors are associated with transformational leadership style: idealized influence (behaviors), idealized influence (attributes), inspirational motivation, intellectual stimulation, and individual consideration.[16] Idealized influence (behaviors) is the trust and confidence a leader builds with followers through personal association. Idealized influence (attributes) is how a leader develops a collective sense of mission and values with followers. Inspirational motivation is promoting a clear vision by the leader to followers. Intellectual stimulation is the promotion of innovation and creativity

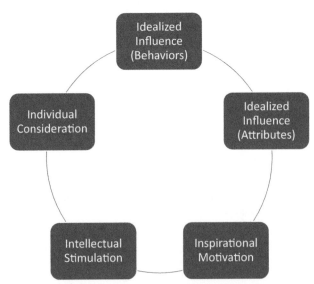

Fig. 4. Transformational leadership factors. (*Adapted from* Bass, B. & Avolio, B (1993). Transformational Leadership: A Response to Critiques. In Leadership Theory and Research: Perspectives and Directions (pp. 49–80. Academic Press.)

among followers by the leader. Finally, individualized consideration is the empowerment is facilitated through the leader by encouraging autonomy and the voice of the staff.

SUMMARY

BSN students are educated using a variety of techniques to facilitate advancement from novice to expert in cardiac care management. Education in the care of HF requires training across courses to support student learning for these complex patients. Leadership strategies are included in BSN training to ensure they are prepared for the care management and disease management needs of this population. Education delivery techniques use classroom, laboratory, and simulation as well as clinical training. This variety of strategies prepares the student to deliver competent and safe care to this population across a wide variety of health care scenarios.

CLINICS CARE POINTS

- Strategies to transition students from novice to expert over the course of the BSN program include didactic education, case studies, role play, and simulation
- Topics taught to students learning about patients with HF include the 3 "Ps" of holistic cardiovascular patient care: pathophysiology, pharmacology, and physical assessment
- Leadership strategies are included in BSN training to ensure they are prepared for the care management and disease management needs of this population.
- Achievement of defined skills can be achieved through clear goal identification, team player, problem-solving approach, determination and grit, methodological and practical approaches, rewards, effective communication, and vision

REFERENCES

1. AACN. Creating a more highly qualified nursing workforce. 2019. Retrieved from: Available at. https://www.aacnnursing.org/news-information/fact-sheets/nursing-workforce.
2. Benner PE. From novice to expert: Excellence and power in clinical nursing practice. Nursing Division: Addison-Wesley Pub. Co.; 1984.
3. AACN. The impact of education on nursing practice. 2019. Retrieved from: Available at. https://www.aacnnursing.org/Portals/42/News/Factsheets/Education-Impact-Fact-Sheet.pdf.
4.. Avallone M, Cantwell E. Teaching nursing students to provide effective heart failure patient education using a peer teaching strategy. J Nurs Educ Pract 2017;7(2).
5. Cooper LT, Deswal A, Fonarow GC, et al, American Heart Association Committee On Heart Failure And Transplantation Of The Council On Clinical Cardiology; Council On Cardiovascular Disease In The Young; Council On Cardiovascular And Stroke Nursing; Council On Epidemiology And Prevention; And Council On Quality Of Care And Outcomes Research, Current diagnostic and treatment strategies for specific dilated cardiomyopathies: a scientific statement from the american heart association.Circulation. 2016; 134:e579–e646.
6. Heidenreich PA, Albert NM, Allen LA, et al. Forecasting the impact of heart failure in the United States.Circ Heart Fail. 2013; 6:606–619.

7. Sadayappan S. Cardiovascular leaders are made, not born. Circ Res 2019; 124(4):484–7.
8. Ariosto D, Harper E, Wilson M, et al. Population health: a nursing action plan. JAMIA Open 2018;1(1):7–10.
9. Agency for Healthcare Research and Quality. (2021) Designing and implementing medicaid.
10. Disease and care management programs. The care management evidence base for congestive heart failure. Available at. https://www.ahrq.gov/patient-safety/settings/long-term-care/resource/hcbs/medicaidmgmt/mm8b.html.
11. Hollenberg SM, Warner Stevenson L, Ahmad T, et al. ACC expert consensus decision pathway on risk assessment, management, and clinical trajectory of patients hospitalized with heart failure: a report of the American College of Cardiology Solution Set Oversight Committee. J Am Coll Cardiol 2019;74: 1966–2011.
12. Jaarsma T. Inter-professional team approach to patients with heart failure. Heart (British Cardiac Society) 2005;91(6):832–8. https://doi.org/10.1136/hrt.2003.025296. Available at.
13. Krówczyńska D, Jankowska-Polańska B. Nurses as educators in the comprehensive heart failure care programme-Are we ready for it? Nurs open 2020;7(5): 1354–66. https://doi.org/10.1002/nop2.507. Available at.
14. Ghasemi MR, Moonaghi HK, Heydari A. Strategies for sustaining and enhancing nursing students' engagement in academic and clinical settings: a narrative review. Korean J Med Educ 2020;32(2):103–17. https://doi.org/10.3946/kjme.2020.159. Available at.
15. Moon SE, Van Dam PJ, Kitsos A. Measuring transformational leadership in establishing nursing care excellence. Healthcare (Basel) 2019;7(4):132. https://doi.org/10.3390/healthcare7040132. Available at.
16. Bass B, Avolio B. Transformational leadership: a response to critiques. In: Leadership theory and research: Perspectives and Directions. Academic Press; 1993. p. 49–80.

Prevention of Pressure Injury in Patients Hospitalized with Heart Failure

Victoria Facquet Johnson, MSN, RN, PCCN[a,*],
Krystal Raphael, MSN, RN, CMSRN[b,1]

KEYWORDS

- Pressure injuries • Heart failure patients • Cardiac surgical patients
- Preventive dressings • Prevention

KEY POINTS

- Skin assessment should be done on every patient in the hospital. Pressure injury prevention begins at every point of entry in the hospital, including the emergency department, surgery, and acute and critical care units.
- Patients with heart failure are at greater risk for moisture-associated skin issues, which increase the risk for development of pressure injuries.
- Nutrition plays a significant part in prevention and treatment of pressure injuries. Patients should follow a diet that promotes protein for wound healing.

INTRODUCTION

Individuals 65 years or older are the fastest growing population.[1] Elderly individuals have an increased rate of obesity, diabetes, and cardiovascular disease. This combination of conditions results in individuals requiring assistance with activities of daily living because of decreased mobility.[1] Limited mobility can lead to development of pressure injuries. Pressure injuries occur when certain areas of the body are unrelieved by pressure. The most common areas of breakdown are found over bony prominences, such as the sacrum, ischium, coccyx, elbows, knees, heels, and ankles.[2]

RISK FOR PRESSURE INJURY

Pressure injury formation is a result of a combination of physiologic events and external conditions. There are many factors that contribute to patients being at higher risk, such as prolonged pressure, "moisture, temperature, age, incontinence,

[a] Traction Department, East Jefferson General Hospital, Metairie, LA, USA; [b] Wound and Ostomy Care, Diabetes Management, East Jefferson General Hospital, Metairie, LA, USA
[1] Present address: 4200 Houma Boulevard, Main Hospital, 6th floor, Metairie, LA 70006.
* Corresponding author. 4200 Houma Boulevard, Main Hospital, 3rd Floor, Metairie, LA 70006.
E-mail address: Victoria.Johnson@lcmchealth.org

Crit Care Nurs Clin N Am 34 (2022) 181–189
https://doi.org/10.1016/j.cnc.2022.02.010
0899-5885/22/© 2022 Elsevier Inc. All rights reserved.

Table 1 Risk factors for pressure injury	
Physiologic Events	**External Conditions**
Skin moisture/incontinence	Prolonged time on operating room table or stretcher
Temperature	Poorly fitted medical devices
Age-related structural skin changes	Immobilization on spine board, after trauma, or after orthopedic surgery
Comorbidities	External friction on skin from sliding down and pulling up in bed
Immobility	
Internal shearing forces	

underlying comorbidities, prolonged surgical procedures, immobility, spinal cord injury, low body weight, medications, and shear deformation."[2(p133)] Shear is an internal force generated when the skin is moving in a direction that opposes another fixed structure, such as the coccyx. External risk factors include prolonged time on the operating room table, poorly fitted medical devices, and immobility on a spinal board[1] (**Table 1**).

When the force or pressure exerted on skin and subcutaneous tissue leads to localized ischemia and reperfusion injury, lymphatic drainage becomes impaired. This causes an increase in interstitial fluid and waste to build up in the body and contributes to the formation of a pressure injury. The time it takes to develop a pressure injury depends on many factors, including individual's physiology and the degree of pressure and shear on the body's tissue.[1]

Approximately 2.5 million individuals develop pressure injuries in the acute care setting annually. Individuals who are elderly and malnourished and experience increased length of stay during hospitalization have a higher incidence of developing pressure injuries.[3] Prevention and early detection of pressure injury are key. Consequently, developing a structured skin care routine using the appropriate products is an essential component in preventing and treating pressure injuries.[4] If pressure injuries are detected early, measures can be implemented to prevent worsening and impact on the patient's morbidity and quality of life.

FINANCIAL IMPACT ON HEALTH CARE ORGANIZATIONS

In addition to potentially devastating impacts to the patient's morbidity and mortality, hospital-acquired pressure injuries can be a financial burden on health care organizations. The Centers for Medicare and Medicaid Services (CMS) no longer reimburses organizations for the treatment of hospital-acquired pressure injuries,[5,6] and they also may reduce overall reimbursement for the hospital. Previously, the national cost of pressure injury treatment ranged from $3.3 billion to $11 billion annually, whereby a single hospital-acquired pressure injury can cost from $500 to $70,000.[3] Presently, the cost of pressure injury treatment may exceed $26.8 billion yearly.[7] Approximately $1.5 billion is spent annually to treat perioperative-acquired pressure injuries.[8] Approximately 60,000 deaths per year in the United States are related to pressure injuries.[9]

PRESSURE INJURIES AND HEART FAILURE

In America, there are 5.7 million people who are diagnosed with heart failure (HF), which is associated with high rates of mortality, hospitalization, and decreased quality of life. Characteristics of HF are "dyspnea, cognitive dysfunction, depression, and pain."[10(p23)] Individuals with HF also have a variety of factors that can lead to poor nutrition and weight loss, including dietary sodium restrictions and build-up of fluid that can interfere with indigestion and decrease appetite. Also contributing to an increased risk of pressure injuries are poor circulation and limited mobility (**Table 2**). An observational study was performed using data from the CMS whereby 15,459 patients with HF were hospitalized at 149 different sites and 24.1% of patients were discharged to a skilled nursing facility (SNF). Characteristics associated with patients being discharged to SNF are "longer hospital stay, older age, female gender, hypotension, increased left ventricular ejection fraction indicating preserved ejection fraction, nonischemic heart failure, and certain comorbidities (history of depression and stroke)."[10(p22)] In the long-term acute care setting, many of the individuals were receiving medications recommended by national practice guidelines for HF in addition to diuretics.

Table 2
Heart failure risk factors for pressure injury

HF Symptom or Issue	Increase in Pressure Injury Risk
Orthopnea	Sitting up to breathe better increases shear
Dyspnea on exertion	Limits activity/promotes immobility
Cognitive dysfunction & depression	Affect mobility and adequate nutrition
Edema in legs	Discomfort when walking and sitting with feet elevated promote immobility
Edema in abdomen	Decreased appetite/malnutrition
Diuretics	Urinary incontinence, increases moisture
Reduced cardiac output	Decreased tissue perfusion and oxygenation

Incontinence

One of the comorbidities that increases the risk of developing pressure injuries is urinary or fecal incontinence. Urinary incontinence is common in heart disease and diabetes in older women. An individual who is incontinent is at a high risk of having skin damage owing to moisture-associated issues. Prolonged exposure of the skin to moisture causes damage. In addition, excess moisture increases the risk of friction damage. When the skin stays moist and there is pressure at the same time, this creates the perfect storm for skin to break down and form pressure injuries.

A mainstay of symptom management for patients with HF is diuretics, which relieve dyspnea through increasing urinary output, thereby reducing preload.[4] If elderly individuals become incontinent on diuretic therapy, this could lead to incontinence-associated dermatitis. Incontinence-associated dermatitis occurs when urine and feces are exposed to the skin for a long period of time. In some community settings, elderly individuals who are incontinent wear diapers. If diapers are not checked hourly and replaced when wet or soiled, the moisture from urine or feces on fragile skin promotes breakdown.

An older misconception in the acute care setting is that patients with acute HF require indwelling urinary catheters to achieve accurate intake and output data. However, organizations are decreasing the use of indwelling catheters owing to the increased risk of developing a catheter-associated urinary tract infection (CAUTI). The external catheter is a device used to manage incontinence without the use of indwelling catheters to combat CAUTIs. Patients with HF who are bedbound or have impaired mobility and are incontinent can benefit from an external catheter to obtain accurate intake and output.[8] Care must be taken during clinician education and product placement. If the external catheters are not properly placed, this could increase moisture in areas prone to breakdown on pressure points for men and women, which could lead to an increased chance of developing pressure injuries.

In order to prevent pressure injuries, a structured skin care routine, including ensuring optimal skin cleansing, drying, and moisturizing with appropriate barrier products after each episode of involuntary loss of urine or stool, prevents the formation of a pressure injury.

Mobility

Individuals who have HF are at increased risk for pressure injury owing to decreased mobility for a variety of reasons. Because of volume overload, many patients with HF have dyspnea on exertion that causes them to limit activity. Edema of the legs can be painful for patients when walking. Sometimes patients are to elevate their legs while they rest to decrease the edema, but this advice can inadvertently lead to increased immobility. Even while in bed, orthopnea may cause the patient with HF to sit up for prolonged periods of time to decrease the feeling of breathlessness. This position increases internal shear from the coccyx bone to the sacral area and thus further increases risk for pressure injury.

Circulation

In cardiac patients, pressure injuries usually occur over bony prominences, such as ears, coccyx, heels, and elbows. The ischemic skin damage is a result of restricted blood flow from prolonged pressure.[4] Individuals who are considered the highest risk of developing pressure injuries are cardiac surgical patients with the incidence rate of 29.5% owing to factors of comorbidities and surgical procedures. The most commonly studied cardiac surgical intervention is coronary artery bypass grafting, which accounts for pressure injury incidences as high as 53.4% in the Cardiac Intensive Care Unit. Cardiac surgical patients with advanced HF who require implantable ventricular assist devices and total artificial hearts are at risk because of a reduction in cardiac function, perfusion, and immobility. By 2030, it is estimated that 8 million people will be diagnosed with HF, and HF will be the leading cause of disability.[7]

Many people with HF also have peripheral artery disease, which contributes to the development of pressure injuries. Peripheral artery disease is the narrowing of the peripheral arteries that carry blood away from the heart to other parts of the body. Pain, difficulty ambulating, discoloration, and ulcer formation are common if the blockage is in the peripheral arteries of the legs. The most common type of peripheral artery disease is lower-extremity peripheral artery disease, which affects blood flow to the legs and feet. If left untreated, this can lead to gangrene and amputation.[11] When individuals have impaired mobility, their body weight restricts blood flow to their arms, legs, and back. The reduced flow of oxygen-rich blood under the skin can lead to skin breakdown. Therefore, pressure injury formation is common owing to the lack of oxygenation in the tissues or blood flow to the skin.[7]

Cognitive Impairment and Depression

Many people with HF also have depression and/or cognitive impairment. These conditions can lead to decreased mobility, adherence to self-care, and worsening nutrition status. Patients should be screened, assessed, and treated. The pressure injury prevention plan should be individualized to include additional education, emotional support, repositioning and mobility support, and nutrition and hydration reminders and support.

Nutrition

Pressure injuries and HF impact an individual's nutrition status, which is an integral part in the prevention of pressure injuries. Within many health care organizations, the Braden scale is the most common assessment tool in predicting pressure injuries in the adult population. The Braden scale is recommended by the National Pressure Ulcer Advisory Panel and has a nutrition component in the scale.[12] The Braden nutrition subscale relies heavily on recording observed or patient self-reported eating habits. Serum albumin levels and subjective global nutrition assessments are superior nutritional predictors of pressure injury development.[12] These findings suggest modifications are needed to address how nurses assess nutritional risk for pressure injuries in hospitalized individuals. When performed, dietician assessments provide the basis for more accurate assessment of nutritional risk and targeted interventions. Nursing professionals should be encouraged to review the dietician assessment and consultation notes, collaborate with licensed dieticians on the HF team, and incorporate the information into a more comprehensive pressure injury prevention and treatment plan.[13,14]

Malnutrition is an independent risk factor doubling the risk of pressure injury.[15] Nutrition interventions aimed at pressure injury prevention may have great potential to affect change. A meta-analysis reported a 26% reduction in pressure injury incidence in high-risk patients when oral or enteral nutrition support was used.[15] Previous research among hospitalized patients at risk of a pressure injury has indicated that patients' knowledge about nutrition for pressure injury prevention is inconsistent. Therefore, patient education on the role of nutrition in pressure injury prevention and strategies for improving nutritional intake in hospital was a key component of the intervention. A simple educational brochure on nutrition for pressure injury prevention was used in the study. Patients indicated the brochure increased awareness of both nutrition and other pressure injury risk factors.[15]

Nutrition and hydration play an important role in preserving skin and tissue viability and in supporting tissue repairs for pressure injury healing. Many acute and chronically ill adults as well as older adults at risk or with pressure injuries experience unintended weight loss. There is a significant relationship between the presence of pressure injury and unintended weight loss.[16] One-third of pressure injuries were attributable to malnutrition.[16] Therefore, nutrition screening should be completed upon admission to a health care setting, and when nutrition risk is triggered, there should be an automatic referral to the registered dietician. Individuals identified to be malnourished, at risk of pressure injuries, or at nutritional risk through nutrition screening should have a more comprehensive nutrition assessment by a registered dietician.[16]

Older adults with HF are at risk for poor nutrition owing to dietary sodium restrictions that further compound a poor appetite. Conversely, patients who tend to consume foods high in sodium have increased risk of leg edema in combination with poor peripheral circulation, and lack of mobility increases the risk of developing pressure injuries.[10]

DISCUSSION OF HOSPITAL PRESSURE INJURY PREVENTION PROGRAM

Because of the increased risk of pressure injury for individuals with HF, a multistrategy approach is warranted to prevent pressure injury during a hospitalization for each patient. A summary of prevention strategies that should be implemented for hospitalized patients with HF as part of this comprehensive program is outlined in **Table 3**.

In addition to patient-specific strategies, a comprehensive quality improvement program should be implemented by health care organizations using the best available

Table 3 Summary of pressure injury prevention strategies for patients with heart failure	
Screening and assessment	Conduct pressure injury risk screening as soon as possible when patient presents to hospital with heart failure Conduct comprehensive risk assessment based on screening results on admission and with any change in patient status
Skin care	Clean skin after incontinence with nonalkaline soap Use skin barrier product to protect skin from moisture Use high-absorbency products for patients with incontinence Use textiles with low friction Use soft silicone multilayered sacral foam dressing to protect skin
Nutrition	Conduct nutritional screening and assessment Optimize calorie and protein intake through meals and supplements in collaboration with a licensed dietician on the interprofessional heart failure team
Positioning	Reposition patients on an individualized schedule Offload all bony prominences and redistribute pressure as evenly as possible Use techniques for patient handling that reduce friction and shear as much as possible (do not drag patient's skin across surface of bed) Decrease head of bed elevation as symptoms of breathlessness allow Elevate heels using suspension device, pillow, or cushion to offload the heel and redistribute weight along the calf Use prophylactic heel foam dressings Promote early mobility whenever possible

evidence. Detailed education should be provided to clinicians on an ongoing basis, including screening, prevention, assessment, and treatment of pressure injuries.[17] Pressure injury prevalence studies and adherence to pressure injury prevention strategies with real-time peer review and reinforcement on education should be performed on a regular basis. Data should be trended over time and correlated with changes in nursing care, products, and equipment such as beds and mattresses.

At a Magnet hospital in the Southeastern United States, the Skin and Wound Assessment Team (SWAT) is responsible for administration and revision of a comprehensive pressure injury prevention program. The SWAT is an interprofessional team that represents multiple units and departments. The SWAT conducts gap analyses with current pressure injury prevention guidelines and literature. They conduct monthly audits on each inpatient unit with real-time feedback and education, quarterly National Database of Nursing Quality Indicators surveys, annual International Pressure Ulcer Prevention surveys, annual evidence-based practice projects, annual house-wide mattress surveys, and ongoing education to team members through orientation, mandatory nursing updates and skills fairs, and unit meetings.

Through frontline staff engagement in SWAT, the following pressure injury improvements have been made:

- One past SWAT analysis of hospital pressure injuries led to the discovery that most patients who developed pressure injuries started in surgery, especially cardiac surgery. Because of immobility in surgery and during the immediate postoperative period in the intensive care unit with multiple comorbidities, patients' skin was at risk to break down over bony prominences. SWAT conducted an evidence-based practice investigation, which included a literature and guideline review along with data analysis and policy gap analysis. This project resulted in the development of a surgical protocol, which began with a pilot study in cardiac surgery patients and eventually expanded to all surgeries and interventional procedures. Patients are screened using mobility and nutrition status, body mass index, unexpected weight loss, and age, in addition to presence of smoking, hypertension, vascular, renal, cardiac, and peripheral diseases, pulmonary disease, history of pressure injuries or diabetes, and a 5-layer silicone border prevention dressing is applied to the sacrum and heels before the procedure. Comprehensive education and Plan-Do-Study-Act performance improvement methodology were used to enhance the new prevention strategies and patient outcomes.[18,19]

- Following a subsequent quarterly pressure injury audit, the pressure injury rate again exceeded the Magnet benchmark. It was discovered through the SWAT's analysis that with the improvement in surgical patients, 92% of the patients with pressure injuries were admitted through the emergency department (ED). A higher incidence of pressure injury was noted when ED length of stay was greater than 2 hours. The SWAT conducted another Evidence Based Practice investigation and created a risk assessment and prevention protocol in collaboration with the ED. The risk factors were many, but included age, altered mental status, trauma, diabetes, obesity, pulmonary and cardiac disease, impaired regulation of body temperature, altered nutrition, hemodynamics, impaired sensation, incontinence, time on the ED stretcher, and history of previous pressure injuries.[20] As part of the prevention program for the ED, soft 5-layer silicone sacral and heel dressings were applied to patients at increased risk for pressure injury shortly after arrival to the ED. Other prevention strategies, such as repositioning regularly and offloading patient's heels, are documented and subsequently crossed over to the inpatient record to enhance continuity.[21] The ED nurses and other clinical staff were educated on ABCS (airway, breathing, circulation, and skin) assessment and provided data on improvement in the pressure injury rate.
- In combination with the implementation of preventive silicone dressings, a new process was implemented to involve SWAT and other clinicians in assessing mattresses within the organization annually. In implementing this new process, 62% of mattresses were changed owing to a lack of supportive surface.
- Documentation of pressure injuries that were present on admission was not meeting organizational standards. SWAT went to the clinicians to find out what barriers were in the way and discovered that the technology was breaking down. SWAT advocated for new technology. Their advocacy resulted in administrative approval and ultimately enhanced admission documentation of pressure injuries.
- SWAT has empowered additional skin champions on each unit who provide real-time feedback to clinicians as an extension of SWAT. These champions also conduct random monthly audits on patients to determine if prevention methods are being implemented optimally and providing just-in-time peer review as needed. Unit skin champions, all nurses, and all patient care technicians received education including case studies of patients who developed pressure injuries, trended data and improvements, information about the cost of pressure injuries, and legal risks that can be mitigated through appropriate documentation about skin.

Because of the hard work of the SWAT, including patient prevalence studies, nursing intervention audits, reviews of the literature, and multiple new protocols over the last 5 years, the incidence of pressure injuries dramatically decreased within the organization. The program has been such a success that the organization was asked to share the pressure injury prevention strategies as a health care system-wide improvement project.

SUMMARY

For many reasons, patients who are admitted to the hospital with HF are at increased risk for developing pressure injury. Some of these risk factors include incontinence related to diuretics, circulatory problems, decreased mobility, malnutrition, friction and shear, depression, and cognitive impairment. Individual patient risk and strategies to prevent pressure injury must be addressed. In addition, hospitals must have comprehensive programs to screen, assess for, and prevent pressure injury. Pressure injuries can have a devastating impact on a patient's quality of life, morbidity, and mortality following hospitalization. It can also have a negative financial impact for the health care organization. A multifaceted approach must be taken beginning with all points of entry to the organization. Frontline team member engagement is critical, as well as education, peer review, and continual performance improvement.

CLINICS CARE POINTS

- Hospitalized patients with heart failure are at an increased risk of developing pressure injuries owing to intrinsic and extrinsic factors.
- All points of entry into the hospital should assess patients to determine if they are at an increased risk of developing pressure injuries. If patients meet criteria, a 5-layer silicone border dressing is placed on the sacrum and bilateral heels as well as pictures taken over bony prominences.
- Team members' input in the development of new protocols and proper education is essential in a successful implementation of a new product and process.

DISCLOSURE

The authors have nothing to disclose.

REFERENCES

1. Boyko TV, Longaker MT, Yang GY. Review of current management of pressure ulcers. Adv Wound Care 2018;7(2):57–67.
2. Brindle CT, Wegelin JA. Prophylactic dressing application to reduce pressure ulcer formation in cardia surgery patients. J Ostomy Continence Nurs 2012;39(2): 133–42.
3. Padula WV, Delarmente BA. The national cost of hospital-acquired pressure injuries in the United States. 2019. Available at: https://doi.org/10.1111/iwj.13071. Accessed September 16, 2021.
4. Holroyd S. Moisture-associated skin damage caused by incontinence. J Community Nurs 2021;35(4):58–64.
5. Black J, Clark M, Dealey C, et al. Dressings as an adjunct to pressure ulcer prevention: consensus panel recommendations. Interv Wound J 2014;12:484–8.
6. Blenman J, Maran D. Pressure ulcer prevention is everyone's business: the PUPS project. Br J Nurs 2017;26(6):516–26.
7. Brindle T. Incidence and variables predictive of pressure injuries in patients undergoing ventricular assist device and total artificial heart surgeries: an 8-year retrospective cohort study. Adv Skin Wound Care 2020;33:651–60.
8. Wadlund DL. Maintaining skin integrity in the OR. OR Nurse 2010;4(2):26–32.

9. Preventing sacral pressure ulcer development in the surgical patient population. 2014. Available at: http://www.smith-nephew.com/global/assets/pdf/products/wound/us/alce-55-0115-use%20brendle%20allevyn%20life%20poster_pup%20in%20th%20surgical %20patient%20pop.final%20approved.pdf on 4/8/2015. Accessed September 1, 2021.

10. Pressler SJ, Jung M, Titler M, et al. Symptoms, nutrition, pressure ulcers, and return to community among older women with heart failure at skilled nursing facilities: a pilot study. J Cardiovasc Nurs 2018;33(1):22–9.

11. American Heart Association. About peripheral artery disease. 2021. Available at: https://www.heart.org/en/health-topics/peripheral-artery-disease/about-peripheral-artery-disease-pad. Accessed September 26, 2021.

12. Serpas LF, Santos VLCG. Validity of the Braden nutrition subscale in predicting pressure development. J Wound Ostomy Continence Nurs 2014;41(5):436–43.

13. Cowan L, Garvan C, Kent C, et al. How well does the Braden nutrition subscale agree with the VA nutrition classification scheme related to pressure ulcer risk? Fed Pract 2016;12–7.

14. Garcia-Fernandez FP, Pancorbo-Hidalgo PL, Agreda JJS. Predictive capacity of risk assessment scales and clinical judgment for pressure ulcers: a meta-analysis. J Wound Ostomy Continence Nurs 2014;41(1):24–34.

15. Roberts S, Desbrow B, Chaboyer W. Feasibility of a patient-centered nutrition intervention to improve oral intakes of patients at risk of pressure ulcer: a pilot randomized contrail trial. Scand J Caring Sci 2015;30:271–80.

16. Posthauer ME, Banks M, Dorner B, et al. The role of nutrition for pressure ulcer management: National Pressure Ulcer Advisory Panel, European Pressure Ulcer Advisory Panel, and Pan Pacific Pressure Injury Alliance white paper. Adv Skin Wound Care 2015;28(4):176–88.

17. European Pressure Ulcer Advisory Panel, National Pressure Injury Advisory Panel and Pan Pacific Pressure Injury Alliance. Prevention and treatment of pressure ulcers/injuries: quick reference guide. Emily Haesler (Ed.). EPUAP/NPIAP/PPPIA: 2019.

18. Reddy M, Gill SS, Kalkar SR. Treatment of pressure ulcers: a systematic review. J Am Med Assoc 2008;300(22):2647–62.

19. Cassendra A. Munro, C.A. Risk assessment using the Munro pressure ulcer risk assessment scale for perioperative patients. Association of perioperative Registered Nurses. ARON J 2010;92(3):272–287.

20. Fagan M. Early prevention of pressure ulcers in the emergency department. New Jersey: Seton Hall University DNP Final Projects; 2010. Paper 10.

21. Faulkner S, Dowse C, Pope H, Kingdonwells C. The emergency departments response to pressure ulcer crisisVol. II. United Kingdom: Wounds UK; 2015. No 2.

Implementing Evidence-Based Motivational Interviewing Strategies in the Care of Patients with Heart Failure

Nicole Judice Jones, MN, APRN, ACNS-BC, CV-BC, CCNS, CHFN, AACC*,
Ana Richard, LCSW

KEYWORDS

- Motivational interviewing ● Care of patients ● Heart failure ● Heart failure self-care

KEY POINTS

- Motivational interviewing (MI) has positive effects on heart failure patient outcomes related to self-care.
- MI can be effectively used by the interprofessional team in the hospital and clinic settings, and it can be effective even in brief patient interactions.
- The spirit of MI uses collaboration, evocation, and honoring the patient's autonomy. Open-ended questions, affirmations, reflective listening, and summarization are skills used to build empathy and elicit change talk with the MI framework.
- MI has the potential to bridge the gap between patient and caregiver goals and behavior modification to accomplish enhanced heart failure self-care.
- Clinicians can consider obtaining feedback to improve their practice of MI techniques for enhanced efficacy in helping patients with heart failure improve self-care behaviors.

INTRODUCTION

Motivational interviewing (MI) is a conversational direct practice technique created by William R. Miller and Stephen Rollnick in 1983, which focuses on collaboration between client and facilitator to enhance one's motivation for change.[1] Miller and Rollnick initially developed MI as a substance abuse treatment practice. At the time MI was developed, many of the treatment modalities related to substance abuse used confrontation and argumentative natured directives to break through the patient's denial of their own addiction.[1] For example, the first step in the well-known 12-step Alcoholics Anonymous model is to admit powerlessness in an effort to motivate

East Jefferson General Hospital, 4200 Houma Boulevard, Metairie, LA 70006, USA
* Corresponding author.
E-mail address: Nicole.jones4@lcmchealth.org

Crit Care Nurs Clin N Am 34 (2022) 191–204
https://doi.org/10.1016/j.cnc.2022.02.011
0899-5885/22/© 2022 Elsevier Inc. All rights reserved.

change.[2] There is evidence that authoritative approaches are actually linked to increased resistance to change.[3]

MI can be viewed as a therapeutic alternative to heavily rooted confrontational techniques by highlighting empathy, patient empowerment, self-efficacy, and patient capacity for change. MI has even been found to be equivalent if not more effective than cognitive behavioral therapy regarding decreasing substance abuse in adults.[4] This method has since been revised, applied, and found effective regarding positive behavior changes with patients in multiple disciplines, including eating disorders, exercise, smoking cessation, adolescent behavioral outbursts, cancer treatments, diabetic compliance, and mental health interventions.[1,3,5–7] If used proficiently, MI can be conversationally applied in the health care setting by multidisciplinary staff to elicit increased patient motivation for self-care specifically for patients with a heart failure (HF) diagnosis.

Motivational Interviewing Use in Health Care

Patients with a chronic illness diagnosis have been found to retain only 50% of clinical education provided to them.[5] This can lead to discrepancies in self-care related to chronic illness. MI is more effective in establishing medication adherence than education alone.[7] Eliciting motivations for change, rather than solely providing education, can lead to more sustained self-care strategies and improved quality of life.[8]

MI can be applied to address specific self-care behaviors for patients with HF, including adhering to daily weighing, fluid intake, sodium restrictions, medication regimens, and monitoring and reporting symptoms. Once the spirit of MI techniques are mastered, behavior action planning can take less that 5 to 10 minutes in a health care setting with a patient follow-through rate of 70% to 80%.[5]

What Is Motivational Interviewing

The spirit of MI can be summarized by three concepts: collaboration, evocation, and honoring autonomy.[1] MI encourages a *collaborative* conversation between patient and practitioner in lieu of directives. The practitioner facilitates and guides conversation with the patient to establish goals and motivation for change. This is done by *evoking* answers from the patient that inform the practitioner of the patient motivation and ambivalence toward change. The practitioner can guide a patient toward change using specific strategies. Ultimately, however, the spirit of MI *honors the autonomy* of the individual to determine goals and readiness. The 4 basic principles of MI are to express empathy, roll with resistance, develop discrepancies, and support self-efficacy[3] (**Table 1**).

Expressing empathy
The first principle of MI is to lead with empathy. Empathy in relation to health care is considered the ability of the practitioner to recognize the patient's feelings and communicate it back to them.[9] This can help validate emotional responses and build rapport. Using empathy is correlated to higher levels of patient trust and patient satisfaction.[10] Empathetic interactions with patients have also been found mutually beneficial and are linked to reduced rates of practitioner burnout.[8]

Rolling with resistance
In the spirit of MI, if patient resistance to change arises during MI intervention, the resistance should not be confronted directly. Instead, deescalation strategies, such as reflective listening, can help the practitioner align with the patient and understand barriers. The practitioner can assist the patient in exploring thought processes without judgment of "wrong answers" or "correcting" the patient.

Table 1
Spirit of motivational interviewing versus confrontation

	Spirit of MI	Confrontational Approach
Collaboration	Practitioner approaches the conversation as a partnership in which the patient is the expert regarding their own motivations and limitations to self-care	Practitioner regards the patient as unmotivated for change and tries to convince the patient to implement self-care
Evocation	Practitioner facilitates conversation linking the discrepancy between patient's desired change and current behaviors	Practitioner assumes patient ignorance regarding risks of targeted behavior and provides clinical education
Honoring autonomy	Practitioner acknowledges the patient's right to establish their own readiness for change. Assists in decision making by providing guidance and education	Practitioner imposes directives based on practitioner established behavior goals

Developing discrepancy
Cognitive dissonance refers to the theory that patients cannot hold 2 conflicting beliefs at 1 time.[1] A change activator component of MI is to promote the patient's awareness of cognitive dissonance in their values. Once a patient identifies their conflicting values, behavior modification can transition the precontemplation to the contemplation phase of change. Developing discrepancy also elicits the use of patient change talk (responses regarding desired change) versus sustain talk (patient responses regarding maintaining the status quo).[6]

Supporting self-efficacy
Self-efficacy refers to the patient's belief in their own ability to change. MI techniques seek to promote patient strengths and help to build confidence in their ability to enact change. Patients who feel unmotivated, or in the precontemplation stage of change, often have negative outlooks on their efficacy regarding change. Genuinely promoting current and evident strengths empowers patients to use change talk and move through the phases of change.[11]

Current Evidence About the Use of Motivational Interviewing in Heart Failure

The prevalence of HF in adults is expected to increase by 46% from 2012 to 2030, ultimately affecting more than 8 million people.[12] A HF diagnosis carries with it a critical need for knowledge and skills to maintain health and avoid decompensation and repeat hospitalizations. It is essential for adults with HF to be able to perform adequate self-care, as they typically spend less than 1% of their time each year with HF providers.[13] Health care organizations have focused extensive resources on patient education strategies to enhance self-care. Although many interventions have demonstrated improvements in self-care, the rate at which patients with HF are readmitted to the hospital within 30 days after discharge remains relatively unchanged at 21.9%,[14] which suggests that there may be more to self-care than patient education for the sake of enhancing knowledge about the disease process and self-care skills. After the inaugural conference of the International Center for Self-Care Research in 2019, Dr Barbara Riegel and her colleagues[13] described 7 outstanding self-care challenges, which can be divided into 2 main themes. One of these themes is behavior change and includes reasons such as attachment to unhealthy behaviors and lack of motivation to change. Potential interventions to enhance self-care behaviors described by the same investigators include enhancing motivation and linking behaviors to the patient's goals. These interventions are inherent in MI.

Recent Motivational Interviewing Systematic Reviews

Ghizzardi and colleagues[15] published a systematic review and meta-analysis of 9 randomized controlled trials (RCTs) conducted between 2005 and 2020 that measured the efficacy of MI on enhancing self-care behaviors among patients with chronic HF. MI demonstrated significant effects on enhancing confidence in carrying out self-care and enhanced self-care management or recognizing and handling worsening HF symptoms, but MI had the greatest effect on improving self-care behaviors needed to maintain stability. Several aspects of MI were described by the investigators as being advantageous for enhancing self-care of HF. These included empathetic relationships with health care providers, supporting self-efficacy, and identifying and resolving ambivalence about effective self-care behaviors that are known to lead to success, but not yet used by the patient. In the 9 studies, MI was conducted in inpatient and outpatient settings, mostly by nurses, in face-to-face and telephone sessions lasting from 5 to 120 minutes each over 1 to 8 sessions. The study showed no significant effect on functional status as measured by 6-m walk test and self-report physical functioning. The investigators recommend that more evidence is needed to establish the most effective dosage and content of MI to enhance HF self-care as well as the appropriate education for clinicians administering the MI intervention.

A systematic review was published by Sokalski and colleagues[16] in 2019, which included 7 studies. They identified the same concern about heterogeneity of the setting, intervention, and dose, as well as the lack of details about training for the nurse providing the MI intervention. Fidelity of the intervention was only measured in 3 of the 7 studies. MI demonstrated improvements in self-care adherence (even for patients with depression), physical activity, and knowledge of self-care. In this review, MI also improved energy expenditure, exercise tolerance, and functional capacity. Key aspects of MI were not well described in most of the studies, but 1 study described reflection, empathy, affirmation, and humor to help elucidate the discrepancy between the self-care behaviors needed and exercised, as well as to enhance the patient's self-efficacy. Sokalski and colleagues[16] shared the same concerns about standardized interventions and training for nurses in the MI technique. They also recommended that MI be included in nursing curricula as an evidence-based method for enhancing self-care for patients with chronic illnesses, including HF. They further emphasized this strategy for advanced practice registered nurses, such as nurse practitioners and clinical nurse specialists, as they may be positioned to use MI across the continuum of HF care for each patient, and thus monitor its long-term effectiveness and outcomes.

Motivational Interviewing and Depression

Depression is a common and important comorbidity for patients with HF. Although published statistics on its prevalence vary widely, it is well accepted that depression can make self-care more difficult for patients with HF. Some MI studies excluded patients with HF with depression. A controlled study by Navidian and colleagues[17] in 2017 chose to focus on patients with HF with confirmed clinical depression when testing the effect of MI on HF self-care. Patients were required to have a positive screening with the Beck Depression Inventory (score >21), as well as confirmation of the diagnosis by a clinical psychologist on examination. The intervention and control groups received 4 sessions of self-care education, but the intervention group's education was based on the principles of MI. The HF self-care maintenance and management behaviors and self-confidence were all significantly better within the

MI intervention group when compared with the control group. This study shows MI can be effective for patients with depression and HF. MI is recommended by the investigators as a potential therapy to enhance self-care behavior change for patients with HF in combination with depression treatment and monitoring of psychological symptoms.

Motivational Interviewing and Readmission with Comorbidities

As discussed previously, readmission to the hospital within 30 days of discharge from an index HF admission is sometimes considered a measure of HF self-care success, but patients with multiple comorbidities present an additional challenge in preventing readmission. The Motivational Interviewing Tailored Interventions for Heart Failure (MITI-HF) trial was an RCT that measured the impact of MI on hospital readmission for patients with HF with a focus on comorbidities.[18] For this study, nurses trained in MI examined the patients' responses on the Self-Care of Heart Failure Index to identify gaps in self-care behaviors before the MI sessions to aid in goal setting. The MI intervention group received an MI home intervention followed by several phone calls and experienced significantly less readmission related to comorbidity after 3 months. Specific predictors of readmission related to multimorbidity were MI intervention, age, diabetes, and hemoglobin. During the analysis of the results in the context of prior studies, the authors find that the promotion of self-efficacy within the MI intervention accounts for the improvement in self-care in patients with comorbidities who are known to struggle with self-efficacy.

MOTIVATE-HF Trial and Secondary Analyses

The motivational interviewing to improve self-care in heart failure patients (MOTIVATE-HF) was an RCT that is important for many reasons.[19] This 3-armed RCT was unique, in that arm 1 included MI for patients; arm 2 included MI for patients and caregivers (administered separately), and arm 3 represented usual care. Another unique feature of this study was the extended follow-up and outcome measurement over the course of a year.

The MI intervention was delivered by 18 RNs who had 40 hours of training in MI in addition to education about evidence-based HF treatment. The MI intervention was initially delivered during a 60-minute, face-to-face session and was followed by three 15-minute phone calls completed within 2 months. The RNs developed empathetic relationships, exposed discrepancy between the patient/caregiver's current behavior and that needed to maintain stability in HF, avoided confrontation, involved the patient/caregiver in problem-solving, and promoted self-care self-efficacy. The patients and caregivers enrolled in the study completed all baseline and follow-up study assessments independently and were prohibited from collaborating. The Motivational Interviewing Treatment Integrity (MITI) scale was used to assess fidelity of the MI intervention. Recordings of the intervention sessions were randomly selected and analyzed to reveal less than ideal technical quality (mean score 2.4 and ideal is $\geq$3) and relational component scores (mean score 2.8 and ideal is $\geq$4).

The investigators cite evidence that HF self-care reduces mortality, decreases readmission, and leads to better quality of life. At baseline, all self-care scores were inadequate (defined as <70). At 3 months, which represented the primary endpoint, the improvement in self-care maintenance scores in the MI arms was higher than in usual care, and significantly more patients/caregivers in the MI arms had adequate scores than in the usual care arm. These improvements were considered by the investigators to be clinically significant improvements, as well. Over the course of the year, the MI arms scored higher than the usual care group in self-care maintenance at all intervals (3, 6, 9, and 12 months), self-care management at 3 months, and self-care confidence at 6 and 9 months. Interestingly, arm 2 (MI for patient and caregiver) represented the highest scores in self-care management and was the only group that was statistically significantly higher than usual care at 1 year. Therefore, MI was effective in improving self-care maintenance over 1 year with or without the caregiver, but self-care management only with the caregiver, which the authors find underscores the difficulty of managing self-care problems and the need for help from others to facilitate the process. The authors emphasize, as others have, that the quality of the intervention brings the long-term measurement of its effectiveness into question and recommend longer periods of MI training and evaluation before implementation of the technique.

One secondary analysis of the MOTIVATE-HF trial examined the relationship between MI and health-service use (emergency services and hospitalization) and mortality.[20] Once again, the importance of the caregiver was evident, as the only arm that showed significantly lower mortality than usual care at 3 months was arm 2, which included MI for the patient with HF and the caregiver. A trend toward lower mortality was demonstrated at 3 months for the patient MI arm, but it was not statistically significant. The investigators conclude that reducing mortality in patients with HF at 3 months may reflect improvements in self-care behaviors. There was no effect of MI on health-service use.

Another secondary analysis of the MOTIVATE-HF trial explored the effect of MI on anxiety, depression, sleep quality, and quality of life for patients with HF.[21] No significant changes were found by the investigators in anxiety, depression, or sleep quality in the 3 arms of the study. Disease-specific quality of life, as measured by the Kansas City Cardiomyopathy Questionnaire (KCCQ), improved in both MI groups at 9 and 12 months, and was best in the patient and caregiver arm. A clinically significant improvement in quality of life measured by the KCCQ is represented by at least 5 points. The improvements in the study were 6.72 to 9.19 points, which included all 3 KCCQ subscores (overall summary, self-efficacy, and symptom stability scores). The investigators recommended inclusion of caregivers in MI interventions for patients with HF.

Interestingly, 1 secondary analysis of MOTIVATE-HF detailed characteristics of patients who are MI nonresponders.[22] The study aimed to improve precious HF resource utilization by identifying patients who are less likely to improve self-care of HF with MI interventions. Risk factors for self-care maintenance nonresponse included taking less medications daily and nonischemic HF. The investigators discussed the possibility that more medications and a history of emergent ischemic events may increase the patient's perception of his risk, and health care provider discussions should aim to clear up inaccurate perception of risk. Risk factors for self-care management nonresponse were living alone and higher baseline self-care management.

Clinical Guidelines and Tools and Motivational Interviewing

MI is recommended in the American Association of Heart Failure Nurses (AAHFN) Position Paper on Educating Patients with Heart Failure to provide patient education, facilitate effective coaching, and help the patient change behaviors.[23] The American College of Cardiology's (ACC) 2021 update to the 2017 ACC expert consensus decision pathway for optimization of HF treatment lists MI as a behavioral support in Table 10, "Ten Considerations to Improve Adherence."[24] The investigators emphasize a shift from compliance or adherence to patient and caregiver activation. The 2021 European Society of Cardiology Guidelines for the diagnosis and treatment of acute and chronic HF recommend MI as an educational approach, which engages patients and caregivers.[25] "HF patients who report more effective self-care have a better quality of life, lower readmission rates, and reduced mortality." The ACC's Clinician Toolkit for Improving Cardiovascular Risk Communication includes a document entitled, "How to talk about risk."[26] This document discusses MI and includes many essential MI techniques, such as open-ended questions, patient motivators, barriers to self-care, caregiver support, and setting realistic goals consistent with the patient's values. The AAHFN Web site has a tip sheet for nurses entitled, "Motivational techniques to promote patient exercise and activity," which also stresses MI strategies, such as emphasizing patients' strengths to enhance self-efficacy, assessing their motivating factors, and eliciting change talk.[27]

There is clear evidence that MI enhances HF self-care and other outcomes, and it is recommended by professional organizations. What is less clear for the clinician is how to practically use the MI techniques in the care of patients with HF. There are several online courses available through various professional organizations and universities. What is demonstrated throughout the literature is that treatment fidelity must be assessed, and feedback must be given to allow improvement in the practice. The MI Network of Trainers makes recommendations through their guidance documents about the key concepts, methods of study with practice checks, peer feedback, or coaching, and go on to make recommendations for organizations wishing to equip their clinicians with this skill on a broader scale.[28] These recommendations include organizational support, a culture of patient-centeredness, openness to learning and change, low turnover and satisfaction, and expertise in performance improvement teams and data utilization. Optimally, teams or peer partners can use the MITI scoring tools to assess treatment fidelity and give peer feedback to improve practice.[29]

Strategies for Using Motivational Interviewing in Health Care Settings

There are 4 specific strategies that are used within the scope of MI to engage in conversation with the patient. These strategies are frequently referred to using the acronym OARS, which stands for asking Open-ended questions, Affirming, Reflective listening, and Summarization (**Table 2**).

Ask open-ended questions

To put it simply, an open-ended question is any question that cannot be answered with a yes or no response. Asking open-ended questions negates practitioner assumptions regarding patient behavior and therefore inherently acknowledges the patient as the expert regarding themselves. This technique allows the practitioner to gain insight to the patient's motivations, desire to change, and perceived barriers. Once the patient's motivations are established, strategic open-ended questions can also elicit the use of change talk, next steps, and self-efficacy statements that reinforce positive outcomes.

Affirmations

Practitioner use of positive verbal affirmations confirms the patient's ability to enact the desired change by highlighting patient strengths. Strengthening patient perceptions of their ability to enact change and overcome barriers is a key element of MI and a primary aspect of behavior change.[4] Affirmations must be truthful and genuine. It is important to remember that strengths can always be identified. Simply engaging in a conversation with the practitioner about desired change is considered a strength. A positive view of one's self reinforces the patient's perception regarding their ability to change.[4]

Table 2
OARS (Open-ended questions, Affirming, Reflective listening, and Summarization)

Strategy	Example	Purpose
Ask open-ended questions	"What health changes would you like to see in the next month?" "What are your health goals?" "What motivates you to make those changes?"	• Establishes collaboration • Explores patient motivation • Honors patient's right to self-determination • Elicits change talk
Affirm	"I appreciate your candor." "That's a good point." "You have already shown interest becoming healthier by engaging in this conversation, asking questions, etc"	• Builds rapport • Highlights strengths and builds confidence • Reinforces the ability to change
Reflective listening	"It sounds like you…" "You feel…" "You're concerned about…"	• Demonstrates empathy • Allows for clarification • Helps patient process their cognitive dissonance • Checks for understanding
Summarize	"Let's recap to make sure I understand…" "Let's go over what we covered…"	• Ties together motivation and actionable steps • Helps patient to overcome ambivalence • Confirms goals for plan of care

Reflective listening

Use of reflective listening in the health care setting can be considered the expression of the practitioner's understanding of patient statements. Reflective listening has been found to be the most notable way that the patient understands practitioner empathy and views this as the most profound conversational aspect in building collaboration.[6] Reflecting the patient's own statements back to them not only helps to clarify practitioner understanding but also offers the patient the opportunity to hear and reflect on their own thought processes.

Summaries

Summarizing what has been discussed helps the practitioner and patient move the conversation to a natural finish and, if warranted, establishes patient-determined actionable steps for change. The practitioner has the opportunity to link all the components of the MI together that will be helpful in realizing change.

Eliciting Change Talk

Therapeutic conversation using MI techniques has the potential to stagnate and become cyclically focused on patient ambivalence if "change talk" is not implemented. Change talk refers to statements elicited from the patient regarding their ability and desire to develop a change plan.[5] Desired behavior changes are more likely if the patient uses change talk in conversation.[5] MI offers suggestions for questioning that prompts patient change talk.

Most notably for health care professionals, the change ruler can be considered an effective questioning strategy to help determine patient's motivation for change in a time-limited setting.[3] The use of this question helps the patient to gauge their desire and capacity for change by asking the patient to rate their belief in successful implementation or commitment to behavior change on a scale from 1 to 10. The change ruler assessment can also be used to elicit further change talk. For example, if the patient gives themselves a score of 2, the practitioner can then use follow-up questions, such as, "What would it take to make that number higher?" This allows elaboration regarding motivations and barriers and can elicit further change talk.

Findings show that when the patients implement change talk it can lead to more consistent rates of change.[6] Listening and reflecting alone do not show causality with change.[30] Examples of change talk questions are as follows:

Evocative questions
What changes would you like to see? What concerns do you have about your health? What are your priorities in regard to your health maintenance and self-care?

Hypothetical change
Imagine you have already achieved your health goals. How would your life be positively impacted? What do you think was the biggest contributor to your success?

Review past successes
What has worked for you in the past when you wanted to make a change?

Double-sided reflection
How has the negative behavior benefited you in the past?

Ruler assessment
On a scale of 1 to 10, how successful do you think you will be in implementing this change? What would it take for that number to be higher?

CASE VIGNETTE AND PRACTICAL APPLICATION

A 78-year-old man is readmitted to the hospital with edema and fluid overload related to HF. He has consumed a high-sodium diet during the holidays despite continual statements that he would rather be at home and desires reduced hospitalizations. The practitioner has previously attempted directly addressing the patient's nonadherence to HF recommendations using authoritative statements combined with education in the clinic following previous hospitalizations without success. The patient continues to consume a high-sodium diet.

It would be easy to conclude that the patient is not motivated to change his self-care habits relating to HF symptom maintenance. Instead, the practitioner decides to implement MI.

Practitioner: "I would like to discuss what healthy outcomes mean to you. What would successful management of your HF symptoms look like to you?"

The practitioner has opened the conversation with a spirit of collaboration. The practitioner is evoking change talk statements from the patient using open-ended questions while simultaneously acknowledging that the patient is the expert in regards to his own motivation and values.

Patient: "I want to stay out of the hospital! My grandchildren are in town and I'm frustrated that I'm missing out on this special time with them. Even when I am home, I can't do all of the things that I want to because my legs swell and I've been getting short of breath."

Practitioner: "That must be difficult. You want to spend the holidays with your grandchildren while they are in town. Your hospital admissions, shortness of breath, and edema have interfered with your family time."

The practitioner is expressing empathy through use of reflective listening by repeating the patient's concerns back to him and clarifying understanding of the patient perspective. The practitioner is also beginning to establish discrepancy.

Patient: "Yes, I'm extremely frustrated. I'm just tired of being in the hospital. I know that I haven't been following my HF diet, but my family cooks so well and I don't want to miss out on the traditions because of my HF diagnosis."

Practitioner: "It sounds like you have an extremely supportive and loving family who are great at making memories. You have a lot of positive factors working for you. What has worked for you in the past when you successfully celebrated a special occasion and maintained your HF self-care?"

In this instance, the practitioner is affirming the patient's strengths and ability to change while eliciting change talk.

Patient: "My wife and I tried different low-sodium recipes and brought our own dishes to the potluck."

Practitioner: "You have already done a great job at navigating special occasions by cooking food specifically for you to maintain compliance and partake in special occasions. On a scale of 1 to 10, how successful do you think you will be in implementing this change again?"

Implementing the change ruler helps the practitioner to gauge patient motivation and barriers to change. This can help the practitioner to determine which MI techniques to implement next depending where the patient is in relation to motivation for change.

Patient: "I'm not sure. Maybe a 4?"

Practitioner: "Thank you for being transparent. Food is an important part of your family's holiday celebration. You want to partake in the traditions by eating and drinking and you also want to stay out of the hospital for symptoms that are exacerbated by not adhering to a low-sodium diet. Change can be difficult. If you want to continue to celebrate with the food your family cooks, then I support your decision. If you want to start thinking of ways to incorporate a low-sodium diet to help you stay out of the hospital, we can talk about that too. What are your thoughts?"

The practitioner is now tying together multiple MI techniques. This example begins with affirming a patient strength. The practitioner then summarizes the patient concerns and cognitive dissonance by developing discrepancy. Using empathy, the practitioner notes how difficult change must be. The practitioner then aligns themselves with the patient's right to autonomy. This is an effort to elicit patient's decision and resolve regarding motivation for change. This example ends with a patient check-in to make sure that collaboration is in effect. If the patient is ready for change, the practitioner can then transition to planning.

DISCUSSION

Health care providers are taught to assess, diagnose, educate, and implement directive plans of care as the experts that they are. Using MI may initially seem counterintuitive to the practitioner's knowledge and skill set. MI is not meant to minimize the practitioner's expertise regarding health care, but rather elevate the patient's expertise. Every patient's motivations and barriers to care are unique. Therapeutic alliance is an essential mechanism of change.[31] Recognizing and communicating with the patient as an equal expert in their health care planning enhances practitioner effectiveness.[32]

The relational essence and qualitative nature of MI have historically proven challenging to measure proficiency.[31] Competency does not always correlate to proficiency.[6] Stronger fidelity tends to be realized with patients who report lower levels of motivation, even if the practitioner is trained to use advanced MI skills.[33] The efficacy of MI has been well documented, but the degree of measured effect varies.[6] This may account for why many studies chose to focus on the feasibility of implementation rather than fidelity.[33] The MITI 4 has been developed as an MI fidelity tool and is now widely considered a reliable measure of MI proficiency.[29] The MITI 4 evolved to assess complex MI skills, including cultivating change talk, softening sustain talk, partnership, and empathy using a Likert scale.[29] The overwhelming suggestion to assure accurate and sustained execution of MI is to implement posttraining supervision with feedback.[34] Supervision and use of the MITI 4 is the most appropriate avenue to ensure fidelity when implementing MI into practice.

Considerations

Although MI can be beneficial and enhance desire to change, there are some controversies to using this technique. For example, the strategies in MI focus primarily on self-determination. This does not take into account larger societal concerns, such as social injustices, generational poverty, race, gender, ability, or insight.[1] This may underscore its relevance as an adjunct to traditional evidence-based HF self-care education and care management interventions, rather than a replacement for them.

SUMMARY

Use of MI techniques can improve self-care behaviors for people with HF. Clinicians can implement the Spirit of MI by incorporating collaboration and evocation and honoring the autonomy of the patient when discussing goals and motivations for behavior changes in relation to HF symptom management. The use of continuing education, peer feedback, and measurement tools, such as the MITI 4, can help to ensure fidelity of MI in the health care setting. Clinicians could benefit from additional research conducted to determine a more standardized measurement regarding the efficacy of MI and behavior change when used in brief interactions in patient care, the optimal doses and timeframes of interventions, and ideal training for clinicians in the technique.

The health care community has recognized the necessity for interpersonal and empathetic communication skills among health care providers and between providers and patients and their caregivers. Many medical programs are now including communication competencies as a requirement for completion of a medical degree.[9] The spirit of MI is effective and can be used by health care providers in a clinic or hospital setting in which time is limited and behavior change is a component of the purpose of the interaction with the patient. There is opportunity for health care practitioners to enhance their patient interactions by including MI techniques in an effort encompass a more holistic, empowered, patient-centered approach to enhance HF self-care behaviors and patient outcomes.

CLINICS CARE POINTS

- Nurses in all settings can consider training in motivational interviewing.
- Key techniques include empathy, avoiding confrontation, developing discrepancy between the desired outcome and current self-care behaviors, and respect for the patient's autonomy.
- Asking open-ended questions, affirmation, and reflective listening facilitate partnership.

- Peer feedback should be considered to refine the practice of MI to improve HF self-care outcomes.

DISCLOSURE

The authors have nothing to disclose.

REFERENCES

1. Walsh J. Motivational interviewing. In: Theories for direct social work practice. Belmont: Wadsworth Cengage; 2010. p. 253–72.
2. Teps of AA. 2021. Available at: https://www.alcohol.org/alcoholics-anonymous. Accessed October 1, 2021.
3. Hall K, Gibbie T, Lubman DI. Motivational interviewing techniques - facilitating behaviour change in the general practice setting. Aust Fam Physician 2012; 41(9):660–7.
4. Blom V, Drake E, Kallings LV, et al. The effects on self-efficacy, motivation and perceived barriers of an intervention targeting physical activity and sedentary behaviours in office workers: a cluster randomized control trial. BMC public health 2021;21(1):1048.
5. Cole S, Bird J. Stepped-care advanced skills for action planning. In: The medical interview. 3rd edition. Philadelphia: Saunders Elsevier; 2014. p. 46–7, 125-144.
6. Frey AJ, Lee J, Small JW, et al. Mechanisms of motivational interviewing: a conceptual framework to guide practice and research. Prev Sci : Official J Soc Prev Res 2021;22(6):689–700.
7. Hogan A, Catley D, Goggin K, et al. Mechanisms of motivational interviewing for antiretroviral medication adherence in people with HIV. AIDS Behav 2020;24(10): 2956–65.
8. Busch IM, Rimondini M. Empowering patients and supporting health care providers-new avenues for high quality care and safety. Int J Environ Res Public Health 2021;18(18).
9. Van Wormer K, Besthorn F, Keefe T. The social psychology of group behavior. In: Human behavior and the social environment a diversity perspective, macro level9. New York: Oxford University Press; 2007. p. 64–5.
10. Buffington A, Wenner P, Brandenburg D, et al. The art of listening. Minn Med 2016;99(6):46–8.
11. Yao M, Zhou X-Y, Xu Z-J, et al. The impact of training healthcare professionals' communication skills on the clinical care of diabetes and hypertension: a systematic review and meta-analysis. BMC Fam Pract 2021;22(1):152.
12. Virani S, Alonso A, Aparicio H, et al. Heart disease and stroke statistics—2021 update a report from the American Heart Association. Circulation 2021;143(8): e254–743.
13. Riegel B, Dunbar S, Fitzsimons D. Self-care research: where are we now? Where are we going? Int J Nurs Stud 2021;116:1–7.
14. US Centers for Medicare and Medicaid Services. Rate of readmission for heart failure patients. 2021. Available at: https://www.medicare.gov/care-compare. Accessed October 3, 2021.
15. Ghizzardi G, Arrigoni C, Dellafiore F, et al. Efficacy of motivational interviewing on enhancing self-care behaviors among patients with chronic heart failure: a

systematic review and meta-analysis of randomized controlled trials. Heart Fail Rev 2021;1–13.

16. Sokalski T, Hayden A, Bouchal S, et al. Motivational interviewing and self-care practices in adult patients with heart failure: a systematic review and narrative synthesis. J Cardiovasc Nurs 2019;35(2):107–15.

17. Navidian A, Mobaraki H, Shakiba M. The effect of education through motivational interviewing compared with conventional education on self-care behaviors in heart failure patients with depression. Patient Education Couns 2017;100: 1499–504.

18. Riegel B, Creber R, Hill J, et al. Effectiveness of motivational interviewing in decreasing hospital readmission in adults with heart failure and multimorbidity. Clin Nurs Res 2016;25(4):362–77.

19. Vellone E, Rebora P, Ausili D, et al. Motivational interviewing to improve self-care in heart failure patients (MOTIVATE-HF): a randomized controlled trial. ESC Heart Fail 2020;7:1309–18.

20. Iovino P, Rebora P, Occhino G, et al. Effectiveness of motivational interviewing on health-service use and mortality: a secondary outcomes analysis of the MOTIVATE-HF trial. ESC Heart Fail 2021;8:2920–7.

21. Rebora P, Spedale V, Occhino G, et al. Effectiveness of motivational interviewing on anxiety, depression, sleep quality, and quality of life in heart failure patients: secondary analysis of the MOTIVATE-HF randomized controlled trial. Qual Life Res 2021;30:1939–49.

22. Stawnychy M, Zeffiro V, Iovino P, et al. Characteristics of patients who do not respond to motivational interviewing for heart failure self-care. J Cardiovasc Nurs 2021;1–10.

23. Rasmusson K, Flattery M, Baas L. American Association of Heart Failure nurses position paper on educating patients with heart failure. Heart & Lung 2015;44: 173–7.

24. Maddox T, Januzzi J Jr, Allen L, et al. 2021 update to the 2017 ACC expert consensus decision pathway for optimization of heart failure treatment: answers to 10 pivotal issues about heart failure with reduced ejection fraction: a report of the American College of Cardiology Solution Set Oversight Committee. J Am Coll Cardiol 2021;77:772–810.

25. McDonagh T, Metra M, Adamo M, et al. ESC Guidelines for the diagnosis and treatment of acute and chronic heart failure. Eur Heart J 2021;42:3599–726.

26. American College of Cardiology. How to talk about risk. In: improving cardiovas-cular risk communications clinician toolkit. 2020. Available at: https://www.acc.org/-/media/Non-Clinical/Files-PDFs-Excel-MS-Word-etc/Tools-and-Practice-Support/Risk-Communications/Updates/5-How-to-Talk-About-Risk-Strategies-for-Success-P13-14.pdf. Accessed September 19, 2021.

27. American Association of Heart Failure Nurses. Motivational techniques to pro-mote patient exercise and activity. 2017. Available at: https://cdn.ymaws.com/www.aahfn.org/resource/resmgr/docs/patiented/Nurse_-_Motivational_Techniq.pdf. Accessed September 19, 2021.

28. Caldwell S, Kemper T, Heberd S, et al. MI guidance documents on understand-ing, learning, implementing, training, and researching MI. 2019. Available at: https://motivationalinterviewing.org/mi-guidance-documents. Accessed September 19, 2021.

29. Moyers T, Manuel J, Ernst D. Motivational interviewing treatment integrity coding manual 4.2.1. 2015. Available at. https://casaa.unm.edu/download/MITI4_2.pdf. Accessed September 26, 2021.

30. Rautalinko E. Reflective listening and open-ended questions in counselling: preferences moderated by social skills and cognitive ability. Counselling Psychotherapy Res 2013;13(1):24–31.

31. Jones SA, Latchford G, Tober G. Client experiences of motivational interviewing: an interpersonal process recall study. Psychol psychotherapy 2016;89(1): 97–114.

32. Pomey M-P, Clavel N, Normandin L, et al. Assessing and promoting partnership between patients and health-care professionals: co-construction of the CADICEE tool for patients and their relatives. Health Expect : Int J Public participation Health Care Health Pol 2021;24(4):1230–41.

33. Small JW, Frey A, Lee J, et al. Fidelity of motivational interviewing in school-based intervention and research. Prev Sci : official J Soc Prev Res 2021;22(6):712–21.

34. Rollnick S, Gobat N. Integrating MI into services: challenges and opportunities. Addiction (Abingdon, England) 2016;111(7):1157–8.

Transcatheter Aortic Valve Replacement (TAVR)

Transcatheter Aortic Valve Replacement Patient Care Improvements; It Takes a Team

Patricia A. Keegan, DNP, NP-C*, Rae Mitchell, RN, MSN, VA-BC,
Christine Stoneman, RN, MSN, CNML, RT(R),
William Shane Arrington, BMSc, CNMT, Angela Spahr, BS, RDMS, RDCS,
Thomas Brown, BSN, RN, Kelby Biven, PA-C, Emily Donovan, NP-C,
Louisa Kalinke, NP-C, Preethy Mathew, NP-C,
Morgan Harrison, RN, BSN, Emily Jones, RN, BSN,
Mary Higgins, MSN, APRN, AG-CNS,
Kenya Hester, APRN, MSN, CCNS, ACNS-BC, Jeanette Gaston, MSN, FNP-C,
Cecilia Mortorano, MSN, RN, NEA-BC

KEYWORDS

- TAVR • Structural heart • Nursing • Pathway • Heart team

KEY POINTS

- Guideline-based practice for the treatment of valvular heart disease recommends evaluation by a multidisciplinary team within the valve program
- Team-based care reduced morbidity and mortality
- Fragmented care contributes to poor outcomes in the treatment of severe aortic stenosis with transcatheter valves.

INTRODUCTION

Team-based health care is the delivery of health services to individuals, families, and/ or their communities by at least two health providers who work in collaboration with patients and their caregivers to accomplish shared goals to provide high quality care.[1] By incorporating multiple perspectives in health care, there is a benefit of diverse knowledge and experience. In practice, shared responsibility without high-quality teamwork can lead to fragmented care and less than optimal outcomes. The high-performing team is now widely recognized as an essential tool for providing a patient-centric, coordinated, and effective health care delivery system.

Emory Healthcare, 550 Peachtree Street Northeast, Atlanta, GA 30308, USA
* Corresponding author. 550 Peachtree Street, Northeast, MOT 1200, Atlanta, GA 30308, USA
E-mail address: patricia.keegan@emoryhealthcare.org

Crit Care Nurs Clin N Am 34 (2022) 205–214
https://doi.org/10.1016/j.cnc.2022.02.008
0899-5885/22/© 2022 Elsevier Inc. All rights reserved.

There is a paucity of data when it comes to the definition of team-based care. Common elements, success factors, and outcome measures are described in a number of scenarios, a widely accepted framework does not yet exist. At Emory Healthcare, our cultural framework, the Care Transformation Model, focuses on transparency, disclosure, shared decision making, cultural competency and diversity, and patient- and family-centered care. Utilization of the cardiovascular team (CVT) within the transcatheter aortic valve replacement (TAVR) program has created an environment of shared responsibilities as well as a focus on the patient.

Team Roles

The historical reference of a physician being the center of health care is no longer an accurate representation of health care. The term "it takes a village" is certainly true when it comes to the provision of care within the structural heart (SH) service. The team is made up of multiple disciplines, administrative and clinical. The patient receives multiple "touches" and therefore care must be seamless to ensure rapid identification and progression to treatment. Delays in care have untoward consequences of elevated risk for morbidity and mortality.[2]

Administrative team

Once a patient is referred by an outside provider, the first contact with the patient is made by our administrative assistants. Patients have several ways to be referred within the system. These include email, electronic medical center messaging, faxes, website pages, text messages to the team, consultations in the hospital, as well as word of mouth. Many avenues for referral care must be given to streamline the process as seen in **Fig. 1**. The team undergoes training with standard operating procedures regarding scheduling, requesting information, patient communication, and insurance verification. The goal of the Structural Heart and Valve Clinic (SHVC) is to have the patient seen in our clinics within 2 weeks of referral. The administrative team has a line of sight to the entire process and direct communication with the clinicians.

Valve Clinic Coordinators & Nurse Navigators: Provision of the right care in the right sequence at the right time requires personnel, resources, and communication among the team.[3,4] Onerous programmatic details within the SH service made program

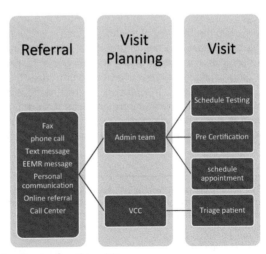

Fig. 1. Pathway of patient referral to visit.

navigation a necessity. To navigate these new program mandates, industry vendors required sites to identify a Coordinator—a role blending clinical and operational expertise, distinct to the research coordinator. The early nomenclature for the position was coined by the industry (valve clinic coordinator (VCC)) and emphasized the procedure (TAVR coordinator).[4]

Navigation throughout the health care system is not a new concept. This role has been well defined in the field of oncology. Operationalization of the role varies on local setting and organizational use. Navigation was created and emerged from the field of oncology in a Harlem community more than 30 years ago.[5] Since its inception, the role of Navigation has been adopted across many health care disciplines with great success in the worlds of transplant, congenital and pediatrics, public health/social work and, in this case, the emerging realm of SH.

Fillion and colleagues,[6] defines the nurse navigator (NN) as an individual registered nurse who uses the nursing process to educate patients, facilitate decision-making and ensure timely access to care via an individualized approach. It is important to note that not all programs use nurses in the coordinator role. Approximately 80% of coordinators hold a registered nurse delegation.[4]

Within our center, we have chosen to incorporate our transplant team workflow into our valve program. Our VCCs care for patients from referral to the procedure. The NN then provides care from the timeframe of procedure to the rest of life. In our center, our VCC position and NN are all registered nurses. Our center felt this was the appropriate degree for the scope of practice to include clinical decision making, triage of patients, patient education, as well as critical thinking. Growth and innovation have enabled Emory's Structural Heart Program to expand its' team beyond a single coordinator as well as the ability to accommodate further role differentiation and allowing for a separate NN position. Emory's format outlines roles divided largely along pre and postoperative lines and have 2 VCC and 2 NN. VCC's are present in clinic and multidisciplinary team meetings coordinating referrals, preop care, education, and scheduling from the first point of contact (initial referral) to the procedure day. NN take over the day of procedure and follow patient indefinitely through the registry period into the first year and beyond, coordinating with referring and local providers to coordinator aftercare. Perioperatively, there is some overlap that exists between the 2 roles regarding preparation for the procedure, follow-up appointments, data collection, and so forth. Most centers have not moved to this expanded model. In 2019, only 2% of surveyed clinicians at SH centers identified as Navigators.[4]

Within the Emory SHVC, the NN role encompasses ambulatory/OP & inpatient settings. In these settings, the NN provides follow-up, operative and postoperative education, staff education and both the internal and external follow-up with the SH team and the patient's local cardiologist or primary care provider. Social services and rehabilitation needs are also addressed alongside recommendations from discharge from the provider and social work teams. Close contact with the patient's referring care team is integral to maintaining the continuity of care postintervention, fostering an environment of collegiality within the health care system, and maintaining a healthy referral relationship. Research has shown that fragmented readmission following TAVR is common and is associated with increased 1-year mortality and readmission.[7] Efforts to improve the coordination of care may improve these outcomes and optimize long-term benefits yielded from TAVR. Using our VCC and NN roles, our SH team evaluates and treats patients from all over the country as well as from outside the United States, so coordination with local providers is critical to ensure evidence-based care, appropriate procedural follow-up, and adequate TVT registry data collection with the goal of evaluating TAVR patient outcomes.

Echocardiology

The Echocardiology team is an integral part of the patient's journey through their SH procedure. Echocardiography is used every step of the way, including assessing the suitability of a patient for a particular procedure, support during the case, and performing echocardiograms postprocedure to evaluate valve and cardiac function. The echo team consists of cardiac sonographers with extensive training that does not end when their orientation is over. The team continually reviews cases and attends educational meetings to ensure that each team member can perform quality studies.

As the sonographers are performing an echocardiogram, they are trained to obtain images per protocol. These protocols were developed using American Society of Echocardiography (ASE) guidelines as well as the requirements of the TVT registry. The TAVR patient journey can begin with the identification of severe aortic stenosis on echocardiogram. Several key measurements are required for the evaluation of the aortic valve. Echosonographers are educated to identify contributing factors to the patient's valvular disease. These factors have implications for the treatment of disease and require further identification. If the sonographer sees any concerns, they have autonomy to collect any additional images. Additional images and techniques may include: going off-axis to image, taking multiple sweeps, using x-plane, or possibly 3D imaging. If the first sonographer has any questions as to the images seen, they are encouraged to seek additional support from a second sonographer. Most of the TAVR cases are supported by transthoracic echocardiography rather than transesophageal. For these procedures, the sonographer first obtains baseline images as the patient arrives in the procedure room. the baseline images assess for pericardial effusion preprocedure, learn imaging windows, and high-level overview to determine any abnormalities that may prevent the case from proceeding as planned. As the case progresses, the sonographer will be asked to check for wire placement before the valve being introduced. After deployment, echo imaging will be used to ensure that there is no increase in pericardial effusion and to check for perivalvular leak. Cardiac sonographers are aware that they are often the first clinician to identify a change in the size of pericardial effusion. The sonographers are encouraged to speak up regarding any potential complications as they are imaging. This team approach helps lead to increased patient safety and procedure success rates. During the closure of the access sites, the sonographer will do final imaging to check for pericardial effusion, evaluate perivalvular leak, and measure aortic valve gradients. Full echocardiograms are obtained postprocedure (if indicated), day 23 to 75 postprocedure, and day 305 to 425 postprocedure.

In highly selected cases, transesophageal echocardiography (TEE) during procedures is conducted by a physician trained in imaging. As in all procedures, the different teams work together and communicate throughout the procedure to optimize patient outcomes.

Cardiac computed tomography

Cardiac structural computed tomography (CT) plays an integral role in TAVR planning with its ability to evaluate the aortic valve, aorta, and iliofemoral arteries to ensure candidate appropriateness, prosthesis types, and optimal treatment approach. Utilization of an ECG-gated multislice imaging approach for the measurement of the aortic valve complex generates high reproducibility with excellent inter-and intrareader correlations. Emory University Hospital Midtown performs all TAVR CT imaging on a high spatial and temporal resolution state-of-the-art 640 slice scanner with rotation speed as quick as 0.275 seconds. The CT scanners' ability to generate a highly reliable depiction of the aortic valve and root anatomy allows for the appropriate selection of the valve prosthesis size. This data is fundamental in preventing potential postprocedural complications such as prosthesis embolization or para-valvular regurgitation.[8]

Every effort is made to adhere to the ALARA (as low as reasonably achievable) principle to ensure patients receive the lowest radiation exposure possible while producing the highest quality images. Software programs should be used to tailor radiation exposure not only by patient size and shape but also by specific imaging parameters selected for each imaging task. Further, dual region of interest bolus tracking and volume scanning capabilities, along with vHP (variable helical pitch) allow for gated and nongated image combination, thereby reducing the patient's radiation exposure and decreasing the required volume of a potentially nephrotoxic contrast agent.

When performing a TAVR examination, some of the key features of the protocol include:

- Obtaining a comprehensive template of measurements, including diameter, area, angle, circumference, and surrounding structures.
- Automated segmentation and centerlines of aorta and aortic root.
- Definition of the 3-point aortic valve plane.
- C-Arm angle display for device placement.
- Ability to plan for transfemoral, subclavian and transapical delivery approaches.
- Creation of stent planning templates.
- Optimal viewing of cardiac valves and calcium.

Our imaging team is comprised of ARRT (American Registry of Radiologic Technologists) CT registered technologists with expert training in cardiac CT. Also in the imaging suite is a Non-Invasive Registered Nurse responsible for monitoring patient vitals pre and postcontrast administration. Patients with SH can expect to be in the CT imaging suite for approximately 45 minutes. Patients are instructed to have nothing by mouth, except for medication, for 2 to 4 hours before the procedure. All patients are screened for contrast allergies and every effort is made to prescribe pretreatment medications to patients with known allergies 24 to 48 hours before testing. Recent serum creatinine values are also required (within 30 days) before the examination; if one is not an available point of care (POC) testing will be performed on arrival.

The valve clinic coordination, nurse navigation, and preprocedure testing processes bookend the patient's day-of-procedure visit and support the seamless intake and transition back to local care pre and postprocedure. The actual day of procedure opens another layer of care coordination and further expands the CVT as many disciplines intersect to provide care according to their specific roles.

Cardiac observation area

The cardiac observation area (COA) is a hospital-based, preparation and recovery unit for patients mostly undergoing invasive cardiac procedures. The COA provides operational and procedural support for invasive cardiology and its clinical staff are responsible for preparing, educating, and recovering postprocedure patients. Because the COA is a highly specialized cardiac care and recovery area, the staff possess extensive clinical competencies and expertise in specialty cardiac care. The COA nursing staff includes registered nurses with previous experience in the emergency room, clinical decision unit, ICU, EP laboratory, cardiac step-down, and medical-surgical areas. Although the team originates from varied clinical backgrounds, all clinicians are trained on cardiac patient care competencies, including but are not limited to cardiovascular disease processes, patient assessment, cardiac rhythm monitoring, prompt dysrhythmia recognition, cardiac medication administration, specific invasive procedure preparation and recovery, arterial line management, knowledge of vascular closure devices, groin management, management of procedural complications, and recovery of patients who have received anesthesia.

The COA clinicians are well versed on the requirements for prepping patients with SH in a timely manner as to not delay their procedure. Preparation includes basic admission information (history, allergies, medication reconciliation), vital signs, IV-line insertion with POC laboratory draws, and a physical assessment to include lower extremity pulse characteristics. Medication administration includes giving buffered aspirin as ordered if not contraindicated. The COA recovers all patients with non-ICU SH before their transfer to the inpatient cardiac step-down unit. The reason for this is to support this unique patient population with specialized, effective recovery care by nurses trained in the management of cardiac procedural complications. Immediate postprocedure monitoring, symptom, and groin management occur in the COA with an expectation to have the SH patient transferred to the inpatient unit within 2-hours postprocedure. Currently, the average postprocedure recovery length of stay (LOS) in the COA is 2 hours and 25 minutes. A 1:1 nurse-to-patient ratio is maintained while recovering SH procedural patients, which allows for close monitoring and rapid identification of critical postprocedure complications that can lead to an extended hospital stay. Recovery monitoring in the first 2-hours postprocedure includes, but is not limited to:

- Hemodynamic stabilization
- TR(radial) band management and removal
- Groin assessment, monitoring, and management
- Neurologic assessment and monitoring

Sedation and general anesthesia assessment and management factors extending the recovery stay beyond 2 hours are typically related to treating immediate postprocedure complications such as bleeding, hemodynamic instability, or organizational constraints impacting inpatient bed availability.

Cardiac catheterization laboratory

Following preprocedure preparation in the COA, the patient is brought to the cardiac catheterization laboratory (CCL) (cath laboratory) whereby the procedure is performed. Care coordination for the SH patient in the cath laboratory is a primary responsibility of the cath laboratory RN. The structural patient population is complex and requires RNs with critical care experience combined with extensive cath laboratory education, and training. A thorough understanding of the patient's physiology and potential procedural complications is critical to the RN's ability to provide excellent care to patients undergoing SH procedures. The CCL is staffed with RNs, registered cardiovascular invasive specialists (RCIS), and x-ray technologists. All of the RNs have experience in critical care in addition to the completion of a comprehensive 4 -month orientation on hire. Cath laboratory nurses are required to have ICU, ER, or CCU experience to provide a foundation on which to build cath laboratory training. The interview process includes screening RNs for current experience managing hemodynamically unstable patients requiring vasoactive drips, airway management, and advanced cardiac life support. Many patients with SH are complex with comorbid conditions that impact their tolerance of structural procedures, sedation, and recovery. Cath laboratory RNs are also required to have a basic knowledge of right and left heart pressures to build an understanding of patients with SH and therapies. In addition, the RN communicates information to the structural team, such as laboratory results, allergies, and previous procedures that enable the team to be proactive in preventing and minimizing complications. The CCL team is able to provide care for TAVR cases under conscious sedation, which requires a highly skilled procedural team. Care coordination with the anesthesia team and COA is also essential to comprehensive patient care during structural cases monitored anesthesia care (MAC) or general anesthesia the anesthesia team is used.

Our CCL uses two RNs staff each structural procedure along with 2 RCIS for both sedation and general anesthesia cases. The RNs are primarily responsible for monitoring the patient, assisting anesthesia, sedation delivery, retrieving and handing off equipment, performing activated clotting time (ACT) point-of-care testing, operating the injector, and rapid pacing. The Registered Cardiovascular Invasive Specialist (RCIS) scrub, monitor, and document procedures. All team members are highly skilled and trained to react to complications. In the event of a complication requiring surgical management, the cath laboratory team is proficient in managing the transition to an open chest procedure until the cardiothoracic surgery team arrives.

The RCIS hold a certification supported by Cardiovascular Credentialing International (CCI), which is a credentialing organization for Cardiovascular Technology. In addition, x-ray technologists are required to either obtain a Cardiac Interventional (CI) certification through the American Registry of Radiologic Technologists (ARRT) or RCIS certification. RCIS and ARRT staff are oriented for 3 months to the general cardiac diagnostic and interventional procedures. Orientation to SH procedures begins after a year of experience in the laboratory. If a technologist arrives with experience the orientation process is designed for that person's skill level, and then advancement to structural orientation is planned.

The cardiology services division maintains a full-time educator who coordinates vendor and physician-led education for the cath laboratory. In addition, staff are tested yearly on medications, rhythm, right heart anatomy and pressures, and coronary anatomy. This education helps keep staff informed of new and changing procedures as well as build a foundation for advanced procedures.

NURSE-LED SEDATION

Appropriately selected TAVR procedures are performed in our cath laboratory with moderate sedation administered by the cath laboratory RN. All participating RNs have been trained in the administration and monitoring of moderate sedation in the setting of patients with SH. Considerations for these procedures rely on the original orientation to SH and critical care experience of managing patients with multiple co-morbid conditions. The SH RNs administer sedation for low-risk TAVRs and follow provider guidance regarding dosing and patient response. Versed and Fentanyl are the primary medications.[9] Hemodynamic measurements (including vital signs, end-tidal CO_2, and heart rhythm), are monitored every 5 minutes by both the monitor person and circulating RN. The patient's response to medication doses is documented and future doses are titrated and administered according to the patient's response. Hemodynamics and level of consciousness (LOC) are documented pre and postsedation along with an Aldrete score. Sedation reversal medications are easy to access, and all RNs maintain competency for administration.

Standardized hand-off was seen as an opportunity for a quality and safety improvement measure.[10] Postsedation patients recover in the COA, and postgeneral anesthesia patients recover in the COA, ICU, CCU, or PACU depending on the patient status. Through collaborative process, a handoff tool was generated to ensure complete information transfer to reduce errors and improve patient outcomes. The preprocedure hand-off is completed between the COA RN, anesthesia, and led by the cath laboratory RN to ensure everything is in place before proceeding to the procedure room. During the procedure, the circulating RN documents sedation medication doses and times, ACT results, heparin doses, vitals, device deployment, access sites, closure devices, vasopressors, or other medications administered during the procedure. Medications for general anesthesia patients are communicated by the anesthesia team to the recovery RN, in addition to procedural information on the handoff tool reviewed with the PACU, ICU, or COA RN. The standardized hand-off created by the CCL has improved communication between the health care teams. The CCL team has the autonomy to recognize an opportunity for improvement, develop a plan for a solution, trial the solution, and then implement the hand-off tool to improve communication. The CCL team has received positive feedback about the handoff tool as an effective communication tool among the patient care areas that recover patients from the cath laboratory.

Bedside Staff

Pre and postprocedure care for the SH patient is provided on specialized cardiac care units. At our institution, we use a coronary care unit (CCU), cardiovascular ICU (CVICU), and 2 telemetry units. These 4 separate units are similar but distinct skillsets to support acuity-based medical and or surgical cardiac care needs. Registered Nurses and patient care associates employed in these areas receive disease-specific training. Competency is supported and assessed through 1:1 preceptorship for periods of 8 to 15 weeks. Didactic training classes include heart failure management, acute coronary syndrome, dysrhythmia, and cardiac device management within medical-surgical or critical care classes. A specific SH curriculum was developed for the care of this population and is presented quarterly to foster knowledge and skill of nurses providing direct care for the SH patient. Nurses and allied health staff are invited to the preprocedural multidisciplinary heart team meeting to provide additional insight into patient care and cases. Our organization also uses a nurse champion program to promote excellence in the care of patients with SH. These nurses receive additional education regarding SH procedures as well as advanced training to manage postprocedure patients.

Advanced Practice Clinicians

American Heart Association (AHA) and American College of Cardiology (ACC) guidelines urge evaluating and recommending treatments for all patients with severe valvular heart disease before considering valve intervention by a multidisciplinary team at a Primary or Comprehensive Valve Center.[11] Our center includes advanced practice clinicians (APCs) as an integral part of the multidisciplinary team. Our SH team is comprised of nurse practitioners and physician assistants to help foster the best patient care and outcomes.

Rymer and colleagues[12] found that APCs provide care that is comparable to that of physicians but with the added benefit of improved patient satisfaction in patients' postacute myocardial infarction. With the role of the APC advancing in both the hospital and clinic settings, APCs are in high demand. The transformation of health care delivery through effective utilization of the workforce may alleviate the impending rise in demand for health services.[13]

APC roles and responsibilities focus on patient care, medical documentation, facilitating referrals and communications, educating patients, families, and medical staff, coordinating with our centers' research involvement, collaborating with the multidisciplinary team for optimal patient and family-centered care, and participating in professional developments to advance our clinical practice. While maintaining role-defined autonomy, under the supervision of a physician, due to state laws, APCs assist in diagnosing medical problems, ordering appropriate diagnostics, developing care plans, and prescribing therapeutics, both in clinic and hospital settings. The structure of our team includes APC inpatient structural service with the physician and outpatient APC in clinic seeing patients in our APC-led follow-up clinic. Additionally, the team provides coverage of our other campuses and performs new patient consultations in the clinic as needed.

A further benefit of the APC on the team allows same-day appointments, telehealth visits, and remote monitoring.[14] For example, amid the COVID pandemic, our APCs have taken a lead role in telehealth visits and remote monitoring along with same-day appointments for patients with worsening symptoms or postprocedure concerns. As well our team was able to pivot to same-day discharge in our patients with TAVR.[15] In summary, the APCs at our center shoulder a wide range of jobs and responsibilities as part of the comprehensive multidisciplinary team and facilitate evidence-based patient and family-centered care while maintaining role-defined autonomy.

SUMMARY

As SH programs increase in prevalence and procedures, the role of the CVT has become an instrumental component of the structural programs. The CVT provides essential care, promotes optimal outcomes, and provides collaborative care for patients and their families. Improvements in CVT inclusion are recommended and are now seen as a component of guideline-based care.

CLINICS CARE POINTS

- Aortic Stenosis has a poor prognosis if not treated in a timely fashion.
- Fragmented care can lead to poor outcomes.
- The Cardiovascular team are essential members of the multidisciplinary heart team.

DISCLOSURE

P.A. Keegan is a consultant for Edwards Lifesciences, Abbott Vascular, and Medtronic. No other authors have any disclosures to report.

REFERENCES

1. Mitchell P, Wynia M, Golden R, et al. Core principles & values of effective team-based health care. NAM Perspectives. Washington (DC): Discussion Paper, National Academy of Medicine; 2012.
2. Campo J, Tsoris A, Kruse J, et al. Prognosis of severe asymptomatic aortic stenosis with and without surgery. Ann Thorac Surg 2019;108(1):74-9.
3. McDonald KM, Sundaram V, Bravata DM, et al. Closing the quality gap: a critical analysis of quality improvement strategies7. Rockville (MD): Agency for Healthcare Research and Quality (US); 2007 (Technical Reviews, No. 9.7).
4. Elizabeth MP, Sarah EC, Kimberly AG, et al. Surveying the landscape of structural heart disease coordination: an exploratory study of the coordinator role. Struct Heart 2019;3(3):201-10.
5. Freeman HP, Rodriguez RL. History and principles of patient navigation. Cancer 2011;117(15 Suppl):3539-42.
6. Fillion L, de Serres M, Lapointe-Goupil R, et al. Implementing the role of patient-navigator nurse at a university hospital centre. Can Oncol Nurs J 2006;16(1): 11-7, 5-17.

7. Wang A, Li Z, Rymer JA, et al. Relation of postdischarge care fragmentation and outcomes in transcatheter aortic valve implantation from the STS/ACC TVT Registry. Am J Cardiol 2019;124(6):912–9.

8. Francone M, Budde R, Bremerich J, et al. CT and MR imaging prior to transcatheter aortic valve implantation: standardisation of scanning protocols, measurements and reporting-a consensus document by the European Society of Cardiovascular Radiology (ESCR). Eur Radiol 2020;30(5):2627–50.

9. Keegan PA, Lisko JC, Kamioka N, et al. Nurse led sedation: the clinical and echocardiographic outcomes of the 5-year emory experience. Struct Heart 2020;4: 302–9.

10. Zou XJ, Zhang YP. Rates of nursing errors and handoffs-related errors in a medical unit following implementation of a standardized nursing handoff form. J Nurs Care Qual 2016;31(1):61–7.

11. Otto CM, Nishimura RA, Bonow RO, et al. 2020 ACC/AHA guideline for the management of patients with valvular heart disease: a report of the American College of Cardiology/American Heart Association Joint Committee on Clinical Practice Guidelines. J Am Coll Cardiol 2021;77:e25–197.

12. Rymer JA, Chen AY, Thomas L, et al. Advanced practice provider versus physician-only outpatient follow-up after acute myocardial infarction. J Am Heart Assoc 2018;7(17):e008481.

13. Woo BFY, Lee JXY, Tam WWS. The impact of the advanced practice nursing role on quality of care, clinical outcomes, patient satisfaction, and cost in the emergency and critical care settings: a systematic review. Hum Resour Health 2017; 15(1):63.

14. Allen JI, Aldrich L, Moote M. Building a team-based gastroenterology practice with advanced practice providers. Gastroenterol Hepatol (N Y) 2019;15(4): 213–20.

15. Perdoncin E, Greenbaum AB, Grubb KJ, et al. Safety of same-day discharge after uncomplicated, minimalist transcatheter aortic valve replacement in the COVID-19 era. Catheter Cardiovasc Interv 2021;97(5):940–7.

Setting a Benchmark for Quality of Care

Update on Best Practices in Transcatheter Aortic Valve Replacement Programs

Sandra B. Lauck, PhD[a],*, Gemma McCalmont, MSc[b],
Amanda Smith, DNP[c], Bettina Højberg Kirk, MSN[d],
Marjo de Ronde-Tillmans, BSc[e], Steffen Wundram, BSc[f],
Nassim Adhami, PhD[a]

KEYWORDS

- Aortic stenosis • Transcatheter aortic valve replacement • Clinical pathway
- Minimalist approach • Nursing • Outcomes

INTRODUCTION

In the first decade of transcatheter aortic valve replacement (TAVR) innovation, clinicians and researchers focused their attention on the development of improved devices, multimodality assessment, case selection, and procedural approaches.[1] These collective efforts resulted in TAVR rapidly becoming established as a safe and effective treatment option for people with symptomatic severe aortic stenosis (AS) with surgical profiles ranging from prohibitive to low.[2] Today, TAVR has surpassed surgical aortic valve replacement (SAVR) as the preferred treatment for AS in multiple international jurisdictions.[3] This accelerated success of *"how we do TAVR"* has now enabled a shift to *"how we care for TAVR patients."* This new focus is driven by early clinical experience, and the pressing need to standardize processes of care to consistently achieve excellent outcomes, patient experiences, and program efficiencies.[4]

[a] School of Nursing, University of British Columbia, Centre for Heart Valve Innovation, St. Paul's Hospital, 5261-1081 Burrard Street, Vancouver, British Columbia V6Z 1Y6, Canada; [b] James Cook University Hospital, Marton Rd, Middlesbrough TS4 3BW, United Kingdom; [c] Hamilton Health Sciences, 237 Barton Street East, Hamilton, ON L8L 2X2, Canada; [d] Department of Cardiology, 3153 The Heart Center, Rigshospitalet Copenhagen University Hospital, Blegdamsvej 9, 2100 Copenhagen, Denmark; [e] Department of Cardiology, Thorax center, Erasmus University Medical Center, Dr. Molewaterplein 403015 GD, Rotterdam, The Netherlands; [f] Universitätsklinikum, Schleswig-Holstein Campus Kiel, Arnold-Heller-Straße 3, Haus K3, 24105 Kiel, Germany
* Corresponding author.
E-mail address: slauck@providencehealth.bc.ca

Crit Care Nurs Clin N Am 34 (2022) 215–231
https://doi.org/10.1016/j.cnc.2022.02.009
0899-5885/22/Crown Copyright © 2022 Published by Elsevier Inc. This is an open access article under the CC BY license (http://creativecommons.org/licenses/by/4.0/).
ccnursing.theclinics.com

In this new clinical context, nurses' expertise in patient-centered care, development of clinical pathways, and change management creates new opportunities for leadership to advance the care of TAVR patients. Nurses are ideally positioned to promote quality improvement initiatives, leverage current evidence, and help recalibrate practices that were often informed by the early era of innovation and surgical blueprints and are ill-suited to contemporary TAVR.

To reach this goal and help prepare TAVR programs for the anticipated need for increased capacity and decreased health service resource utilization, continuous quality improvement warrants close scrutiny of all aspects of patients' journey of care, from referral to follow-up across systems of care. The objective of this review is to outline current evidence that supports the adoption of best TAVR practices and highlight opportunities for nurses to be champions of change to improve the care of patients with valvular heart disease.

DISCUSSION

The goal of TAVR care is to enable patients to safely return home after a seamless and uncomplicated hospital admission to derive the survival and quality-of-life benefits of the procedure. From patients' perspective, transitions from their preprocedure assessment pathway and procedure planning, to their periprocedure experience, and finally to their postprocedure care represent a single journey of care.[5] As such, the adoption of best TAVR practices must encompass a single clinical pathway inclusive of all time points to improve transitions of care and multidisciplinary collaboration.[1]

Preprocedure Best Practices

The central role of the transcatheter aortic valve replacement coordinator

The complexity of referral processes and the assessment pathway create unique challenges for patients with AS referred for treatment. Similarly, cardiac programs require efficient processes to manage communication with referring and procedure physicians, facilitate multidisciplinary consultations, diagnostic imaging, and treatment recommendations, support patient education and shared decision making (SDM), and ensure early discharge and procedure planning.[6] Although titles differ between programs and across international regions, the TAVR Nurse Coordinator has emerged as a pivotal member of the Heart Team to address this issue. Widely endorsed by international guidelines, this role has been integrated unevenly in different regions, with an early adoption in the United States, Canada, United Kingdom, and Australia, and growing or emerging interest in European countries and Asia. Nurses are well suited to excelling in the role, given the requirements for comprehensive and cardiac clinical assessment skillset, patient teaching, leadership, and communication.[7,8]

Although the responsibilities of the TAVR Nurse Coordinator differ across programs, most clinicians focus their work on program leadership and coordination, facilitation of patient-focused processes of care, and fostering effective communication pathways. For patients and their families, the Coordinator acts as a case manager who can individualize communication, planning, and teaching; for programs, benefits span centralized coordination and close collaboration with implanting physicians, diagnostic imaging departments, procedure rooms and in-patient units, research services, and administration. Essential competencies and core responsibilities are summarized in **Table 1**.

Measurement of frailty

The multimodality assessment to inform patients' eligibility and suitability for TAVR requires diagnostic imaging (eg, transthoracic echocardiography, cardiac angiography,

Table 1	
Competencies and responsibilities of the transcatheter aortic valve replacement nurse coordinator	
Competencies and Core Knowledge	**Responsibilities**

1. Expertise in cardiovascular care:
  • Cardiovascular nursing
  • Specialized knowledge of valvular heart disease
  • Specialized knowledge of TAVR
2. Specialized knowledge of providing care for patients with aortic stenosis:
  • Complex heart disease, multiple comorbidities, and frailty
3. Clinical assessment skills:
  • Comprehensive cardiovascular assessment
  • Assessment of frailty and functional status
4. Patient and family education:
  • Assessment of learning needs to individualize teaching
  • Patient and family teaching skills
  • Conduct of shared decision making
5. Coordination of complex processes of care:
  • Organizational skillset to develop and individualize assessment and procedure planning pathways
6. Clinical leadership:
  • Leadership skills to contribute to the Heart Team
  • Administrative leadership to develop program efficiencies
	1. Program leadership:
	  • Serves as essential and central member of the Heart Team
	  • Supports and leads TAVR program development
	  • Participates in program evaluation and quality improvement to improve outcomes
	2. Facilitation of patient-focused processes of care:
	  • Develops seamless and patient-centered processes and clinical pathways
	  • Develops evaluation pathways, including diagnostic testing and functional assessment
	  • Conducts clinical triage and wait-list management
	  • Case manages urgent in-patients and interhospital referrals
	  • Facilitates referrals to subspecialty consultants
	  • Facilitates and contributes to multidisciplinary, treatment decision making
	  • Coordination of procedure planning, admission, and follow-up
	3. Development of communication pathways:
	  • Conducts patient and family education and promotes shared decision making
	  • Leads communication with the Heart Team
	  • Facilitates communication with administration for planning purposes

computed tomography), cardiology and cardiac surgery consultations, and specialized referrals (eg, geriatric medicine, nephrology). Nurses' expertise in the specialized assessment and management of frailty, functional and/or cognitive decline can significantly strengthen a wholistic approach to multidisciplinary treatment recommendation.[9] Frailty is a complex health state that differs from aging; it is an age-related, multisystem syndrome that increases health vulnerabilities when exposed to stressors that increase the risk of functional decline and other adverse events.[10] Frailty is associated with mortality, morbidity, and quality of life after TAVR, and with processes such as length of stay and health service utilization.[11,12] The advanced age of most patients with AS warrants a criteria-driven assessment of frailty and function in higher-risk patients who may not derive the benefits of TAVR, who may require a more in-depth geriatric assessment, and/or when the anticipated procedure planning and recovery trajectory present significant challenges to achieve a good outcome.

Table 2
Commonly used instruments to measure frailty in patients with aortic stenosis

Instrument	Details of Measurement
Fried Scale[43]	*Captures core phenotypic domains:* • Slowness • Weakness • Low physical activity • Exhaustion • Shrinking (unintentional weight loss)
Short Physical Performance Battery[44]	*Captures slowness, weakness, and balance; measured by timed physical performance tests:* • Gait speed • Chair rises • Tandem balance
Essential Frailty Toolset[12]	*Developed to predict mortality after SAVR/TAVR using phenotypic domains:* • Chair rises • Cognitive status (MiniCog: short-term memory and orientation; clock drawing test) • Hemoglobin • Albumin
Clinical Frailty Scale[45]	*Captures clinicians' assessment of accumulated deficits including:* • Presence of terminal illness • Activities of daily living • Instrumental activities of daily living • Chronic health conditions • Patient-reported health status and activities
Rotterdam Frailty Index[46]	*Captures clinicians' assessment of 38 accumulated deficits, including:* • Functional status • Health conditions • Cognition • Mood

There is no consensus on the standardized measurement of frailty in patients with AS.[13] Upward of 20 tools are available and used across programs; the most commonly used instruments in TAVR programs are outlined in **Table 2**.

Patient education

Most TAVR programs can be classified as "procedure-focused" programs: patients are referred by their cardiologist, internist, or other health care provider for assessment of eligibility; episodic care focuses on the short period of admission and ends at the time of follow-up. To match this mandate, the following outlines some key components of the patient education imperatives for TAVR patients:

1. Shared decision-making: SDM is a bidirectional process between patients and clinicians that enables an information exchange, and treatment decisions that consider patients' informed preferences and allows them to participate in choosing the right treatment option. It is not solely patient education. SDM acknowledges equally important forms of expertise to achieve quality decisions: the clinician's expertise, based on knowledge of the condition, prognosis, treatment, options,

and possible outcomes, and the patient's expertise, informed by the impact of their health condition on their daily life, values, and preferences for the possible outcomes.[14] Increasingly, TAVR programs are embracing SDM to ensure patients can make a high-quality decision, especially in light of the emerging equipoise between SAVR and TAVR.[15] Patient decision aids (PDAs) are tools to support SDM; PDAs for AS have been published by American and European agencies to strengthen the adoption of SDM and patient empowerment to participate in their treatment decision.

2. Streamlined assessment pathway: Information about the TAVR assessment pathway must include information about the sequence, scheduling and details of diagnostic imaging requirements, and the expected consultations. The COVID-19 pandemic forced and accelerated the adoption of virtual health platforms to minimize patients' exposure to the hospital environment and further highlighted the imperative need for a streamlined assessment pathway.[4] Additional education may be required to prepare patients for telemedicine consultations, including coaching to successfully connect, accommodations in the case of auditory, visual, or other impairments, and clarity of expectations. Importantly, there may be opportunities to streamline assessment requirements based on clearly defined risk criteria to accelerate access to timely and efficient care. **Fig. 1** illustrates components of the accelerated and routine assessment pathways implemented to facilitate the transition to virtual care in TAVR programs.

3. Preparing for the TAVR clinical pathway: Successful safe and early discharge home hinges on early discharge planning and consistent communication about goals of care from all health care providers at every contact time with patients. This "united front" of uniform communication, inclusive of written resources and clinical interactions with nursing and medicine, is pivotal to avoid confusion, help patients and families prepare "their" discharge plan and availability of social support, manage expectations, and anticipate the important role they play as partners to optimize their outcomes. Key messages for patient and family education must reflect these stated goals (**Box 1**).

4. Early discharge planning: The TAVR Nurse Coordinator plays an important role in coaching patients to prepare for discharge. Effective individualized discharge planning begins before admission to ensure safe transition home. Although the TAVR trajectory of care is standardized and highly predictable,[16] patients who present with unique health vulnerabilities and social determinants of health may benefit from the development of an adapted discharge plan to improve their outcomes and experiences.

Key take-away messages to adopt preprocedure best practices

- The TAVR Nurse Coordinator plays a pivotal role to optimize patients' pathway, communication, and program efficiencies.

- The standardized measurement of frailty augments assessment findings and informs treatment decisions.

- A comprehensive patient education strategy is essential to establish a close partnership with patients.

- Early discharge planning is an effective intervention to facilitate early and safe transition home.

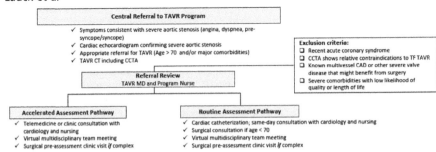

Fig. 1. Vancouver accelerated TAVR assessment pathway adapted for COVID-19.[4] CAD, coronary artery disease; CCTA, Coronary Computed Tomography Angiography; CT, computed tomography; TF, Transfemoral.

Box 1
Key messages for transcatheter aortic valve replacement preprocedure patient and family education

Goal #1: Maximize patients' pre-TAVR conditioning and reduce risks of complications
- Importance of mobilization and physical functioning
- "Stay as active as you can. Ask your regular doctor about what level of activity is best for you."
- Individualized medical referrals
- "The TAVR Clinic nurse or doctors may want you to see other medical specialists."
- Discharge planning: Endocarditis prophylaxis
- "Book an appointment with your dentist."

Goal #2: Develop a discharge plan before admission and set patient/family expectations
- The TAVR journey of care is predictable; standard/goal of care is safe next-day discharge home
- "Our goal is for you to go home the day after your procedure."
- Early mobilization and avoidance of deconditioning are priority activities while in hospital
- "Our goal is for you to walk and do basic activities on the day of your procedure, and to go home the next day."
- Discharge planning requires family coordination
- "Speak with your family about your Going Home Plan."

Goal #3: Facilitate seamless admission and patient safety on day of procedure
- Set expectations of same-day admission
- "Most people come to hospital the morning of the procedure. We let you know what time you should arrive."

Goal #4: Set expectations about periprocedure experience
- TAVR is a minimalist procedure that is more akin to a "big angiogram" than open heart surgery
- The default anesthesia strategy is local anesthesia with light sedation
- TAVR is a short procedure

Goal #5: Set expectations about postprocedure experience and early mobilization
- Postprocedure mobilization after 4- to 6-hour bedrest
- Importance of early and frequent mobilization
- "Our goal is for you to have two short walks on the evening of the procedure."
- Patient comfort and avoidance of opioids
- "Most people who have TAVR do not have a lot of pain. We will check with you to make sure you are comfortable."

Goal #6: Set expectations for next-day discharge and safe transition home
- Target length of stay is next-day discharge
- Safe transition home
- "Once at home, your priorities are to recover safely, rest, get back to your regular activities, and do a bit more every day."

Periprocedure Best Practices

The arc of the development and refining of the TAVR procedure started with the earliest innovation days in the cardiac catheterization laboratory with "interventional cardiology-like" practices.[17] Early clinical trial practices evolved to the adoption of a surgical template to promote patient safety and anticipate the "what ifs" complication scenarios. Most recently, there is increasing evidence that the early vision of a truly minimally invasive and standardized approach is safe, feasible, and efficient.[16] Periprocedure best practices include the adoption of a streamlined approach matched to contemporary technology and evidence, and the development of nursing competencies that are uniquely adapted to the needs of TAVR patients.

Minimalist transcatheter aortic valve replacement

The transition from historical practices primarily informed by cardiac surgery models to more streamlined contemporary TAVR practices continues to evolve. The definition of what constitutes a minimalist approach remains disputed.[18] Important aspects include procedure location, anesthesia strategy, and use of invasive equipment.

1. Procedure location: The rapid expansion of the availability of hybrid operating rooms equipped with high-quality imaging and hemodynamic monitoring equipment provided operators with an effective environment to achieve excellent periprocedure outcomes. This tailored space was endorsed in early guidelines as the optimal setting and became a standard of care in most North American programs and other international programs. Increasingly, the cardiac catheterization laboratory is becoming an appropriate or even preferred space for most TAVR procedures. Careful planning, staff training, and emergency preparedness through simulation training can enable programs to significantly increase their periprocedure capacity, reduce the intensity of operating room resource use, and decrease costs without compromising patient safety.[19] In addition, the intrinsic "nimbleness" of the cardiac catheterization laboratory to accommodate the scheduling of urgent in-patients, and its integration in cardiac service lines offer important operational advantages to improve access to care.
2. Anesthesia strategy: There is clinical interest in selecting an anesthesia strategy that aligns with goals of care of contemporary TAVR.[20] In light of current evidence, these goals include the following:
   - Patient comfort and experience
   - Capacity to easily communicate with patients during the procedure as required
   - Hemodynamic stability
   - Readiness for mobilization within 4 to 6 hours after the end of the procedure
   - Postprocedure transfer of a consistently stable patient with a predictable recovery

To this end, the use of local anesthesia with or without light sedation, or conscious sedation has been reported as safe and effective options for most TAVR patients.[21] Potential advantages of the avoidance of general anesthesia include minimal disruptions to hemodynamic status, improved ability to detect early warnings of complications, prevention of delirium, accelerated reconditioning and predictable time to mobilization, and shorter procedure times. An open visual field between the patient, the anesthesiologist, and the implanting team is particularly effective to promote communication.

To maintain patient safety, periprocedure must retain the ability to convert to general anesthesia, obtain periprocedure imaging within 5 minutes, or initiate femoral-femoral hemodynamic support within 10 minutes. Collaboration consensus agreements between medical and nursing disciplines and regular multidisciplinary simulation training exercises can promote a culture of quality and patient safety, while recalibrating practices to improve care.

3. Best use of invasive monitoring lines: In contemporary TAVR, the avoidance of central venous or urinary catheters is widely accepted across multiple programs and regions.[22] Patient skin preparation and draping aligned with interventional cardiology practice instead of the more extensive practices of cardiac surgery are in keeping with contemporary TAVR. These practices also convey an important message to the patient that the team is conducting a minimalist procedure, and not cardiac surgery. The avoidance of surgical draping and the systematic opening of cardiac surgery instruments have significant cost savings implications. Implanting physicians' systematic use of ultrasound-guided sheath insertion technique and the monitoring of activated clotting time with partial reversal of anticoagulation at the end of the procedure can significantly improve postprocedure hemostasis and contribute to early mobilization. Last, the timely removal of the temporary pacemaker if used at the time of valve deployment in the absence of new conduction delays can further facilitate a rapid return to baseline status and reduce the requirements for postprocedure critical care.

Periprocedure models of nursing care

Multiple factors influence the models of periprocedure nursing staffing models, including procedure room location (operating room or cardiac catheterization laboratory), primary implanting physicians' specialty (interventional cardiology or cardiac surgery), program historical practice, and competing hospital demands. The expertise of operating room nurses prioritizes the asepsis imperatives of valve implantation, assistance with anesthesia, and management of emergency strategy. Similarly, the expertise of the cardiac catheterization team with transcatheter techniques and invasive hemodynamic monitoring, and their competencies in the setting of emergency percutaneous coronary intervention are well suited to the needs of a safe TAVR procedure. The required ratio of distribution of these skillsets remains disputed; nevertheless, TAVR increasingly requires a "hybrid model of staffing" to ensure the availability of the required competencies.[23] The contributions of operating room and interventional cardiology nursing competencies to augment the unique requirements of periprocedure TAVR nursing, and an example of periprocedure staffing model, are illustrated in **Fig. 2**.

Importantly, change in management strategies, communication, education and training, and practice leadership is essential to achieve role clarity and satisfactory selective cross-training of competencies and attend to the challenges of "merging" distinct areas of nursing practice and expertise.[24] Careful attention to equipping nurses to participate in emergency intervention planning and simulation training should focus on emergency vascular repair, percutaneous coronary intervention, management of severe hemodynamic instability and pericardial tamponade, and conversion to open heart surgery.

Key take-away messages to adopt periprocedure best practices

- TAVR can be safely performed in a cardiac catheterization laboratory with close scrutiny of all aspects of the procedure.

- The selection of anesthesia strategies for TAVR should reflect the goals of care.

- The avoidance of invasive lines, the adoption of best practices to avoid vascular injury, and the rapid removal of the temporary pacemaker when appropriate are effective strategies to prepare patients for rapid reconditioning.

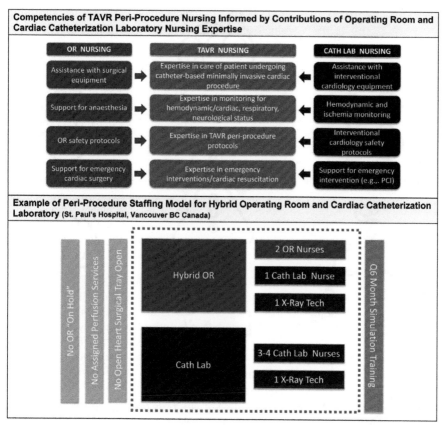

Fig. 2. Conceptual illustration of periprocedure TAVR nursing competencies and example of staffing model. CATH LAB, cardiac catheterization laboratory; OR, operating room; PCI, percutaneous coronary intervention.

Postprocedure Best Practices

Procedural success must be followed by the same degree of excellence in postprocedure care aimed at helping patients to return home safely and early, without sustaining any in-hospital complications or need for readmission, to enjoy the survival and quality-of-life benefits of their new valve. To this end, postprocedure nurses play an essential role in the TAVR clinical pathway to facilitate patients' rapid reconditioning and safe discharge.[25] The early recognition of potential complications associated with TAVR, and the significant risks associated with the hospitalization of the primarily older AS patient population warrant a standardized postprocedure pathway to achieve these goals of care.

"The Big 5": Monitoring for Potential Complications after Transcatheter Aortic Valve Replacement

Contemporary TAVR patients achieve outstanding outcomes, including rapid and significant improvement in quality of life, and risk of 30-day mortality that is as low as less than 0.5%. Device modification, lower profile systems, use of computed tomography sizing, and increased operator experience have contributed to substantial reduction in

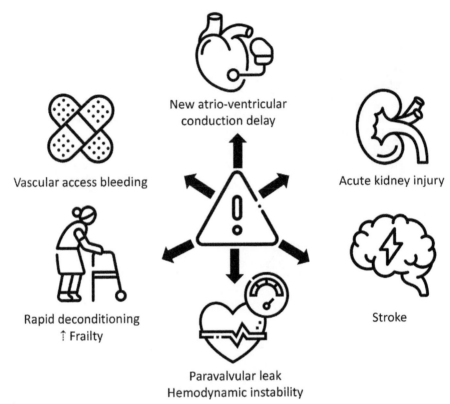

Fig. 3. Major in-hospital complications associated with TAVR (*From* Grube E, Sinning JM. The "big five" complications after transcatheter aortic valve replacement: do we still have to be afraid of them? *JACC Cardiovasc Interv* 2109;12(4):370 to 372)

most complications.[26] Nevertheless, clinical awareness of these adverse outcomes and close monitoring remain essential to mitigate risks and ensure patients have the best possible outcomes.[27] The following important, albeit increasingly infrequent, complications require early recognition and timely and effective treatment (**Figs. 3 and 4**).

Stroke

Different mechanisms and potential contributing factors, including patients' demographics, clinical characteristics, and procedural factors, can contribute to the risk of stroke. Early stroke is considered to be related to particle embolization.[28] Embolic neurologic events can range from a minor transient ischemic attack to a major event causing permanent disability or death. Overall, recent clinical trials and large registry observational studies report stroke rates that continue to decrease.[29] The use of cerebral embolic protection devices remains under evaluation to reduce the risk of stroke.[30] A comprehensive neurologic assessment on admission, and in conjunction with vital signs and vascular access checks, should screen the patient for (1) facial symmetry or changes from baseline when smiling, (2) speech characteristics and presence of slurring, and (3) asymmetrical weakness, numbness, and/or drift when arms are raised. The acronym FAST (Face drooping; Arm weakness; Speech difficulty;

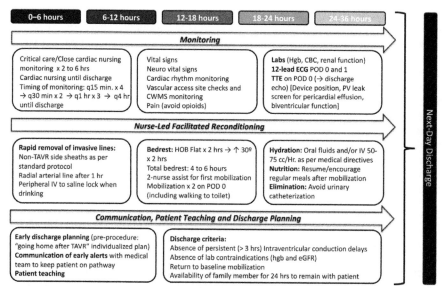

Fig. 4. Summary of TAVR postprocedure nursing protocol.[25] CBC, complete blood count; CWMS, colour, warmth, movement and sensitivity; ECG, electrocardiogram; Hgb, hemoglobin; HOB, head of bed; IV, intravenous; POD, post-operative day; PV, paravalvular; TTE, transthoratcic echocardiogram. (*From* Lauck SB, Sathananthan J, Park J, et al. Post-procedure protocol to facilitate next-day discharge: Results of the multidisciplinary, multimodality but minimalist TAVR study. *Catheterization and Cardiovascular Interventions.* 2020;96(2):450 to 458. https://onlinelibrary.wiley.com/doi/abs/10.1002/ccd.28617. https://doi.org/10.1002/ccd.28617.)

Time to call for help) is an easy guiding reference to conduct a preliminary standardized assessment.

Paravalvular leak

As the native or failed surgical valve is not removed in TAVR, suboptimal placement of the device with incomplete sealing of the annulus, incomplete apposition of the valve stent frame owing to the calcification of the annulus and/or leaflets, or undersizing of the device can cause the onset of paravalvular leak between the device and the annulus.[31] This can cause severe aortic regurgitation and hemodynamic instability. Nurses should anticipate the need for urgent echocardiography and possibly angiography to confirm device function and establish a plan of care. Vasoactive or mechanical support may be needed in the setting of severe instability.

Acute kidney injury

Although there is increasing awareness and strategies to limit periprocedure contrast dye exposure, some TAVR patients remain at higher risk for acute kidney injury (AKI) because of their preexisting renal dysfunction, atherosclerotic vascular disease, advanced age, and/or high frailty.[32] The onset of AKI is associated with significant morbidity and mortality.[33] Close monitoring of periprocedure contrast use, renal function, and rapid resumption of normal hydration can effectively reduce patients' risk and promote an accelerated return to baseline renal function.

New conduction delay

The close proximity between the aortic valve and the conduction system is the primary reason the TAVR device can cause a mechanical insult to the conduction tissue, including various degrees of edema, hematoma, and ischemia.[34] The subsequent development of a high-degree atrioventricular block may require the implantation of a new permanent pacemaker, whereas the new onset of a left bundle branch block may be associated with increased mortality and need for pacemaker.[35] In the immediate postprocedure period, TAVR patients require continuous cardiac monitoring as nurses stay alert for the risk of electrocardiographic changes, especially in atrioventricular conduction (ie, measurement of P-R interval). Increasingly, TAVR programs are endorsing continuity of medical care and the adoption of standardized approaches to the management of new conduction delays to improve outcomes and reduce the risks of pacemaker without compromising patient safety.[25]

Bleeding

The incidence of vascular injuries continues to improve with the availability of smaller sheath sizes, flexible delivery systems, computed tomography imaging of the peripheral vasculature, and operator experience.[36] In addition, periprocedure best practices described in the previous section significantly increase the likelihood that most patients will have a predictably stable vascular access site and will achieve timely hemostasis. Standardized and expert assessment of potential bleeding (including in the retrosternal location) is an essential nursing intervention to ensure early identification and treatment. There are on-going efforts to define and measure the range of bleeding and vascular injury complications to drive quality improvement.[37]

Standardized Postprocedure Clinical Pathway

The postprocedure care of TAVR patients evolved from earlier protocols informed by cardiac surgery to the increasing adoption of contemporary standardized and streamlined practices based on new evidence. In most programs, TAVR nursing care is now well established and integrated in practice; given the low rates of complications and the predictability of patients' journey, this group of patients has become somewhat "less special" over time and now requires substantially fewer health care resources during their early in-hospital recovery. Research supports the transition of historical postprocedure admission to a critical care unit to the preferred use of cardiac telemetry ward for most patients, and the safety and feasibility of next-day discharge home.[38] This recalibration of nursing practices and resources continues to warrant excellent cardiovascular nursing care, albeit not always critical care nursing, that focuses on close monitoring, nurse-led accelerated reconditioning, and communication, patient teaching, and criteria-driven safe discharge home. A standardized TAVR postprocedure clinical pathway provides guidance for nurses to focus on priorities of care.[25]

Monitoring

The assessment of vital signs, cardiac rhythm, neurologic status, vascular access site, and pain/discomfort requires an intensive period of close observation in the immediate postrecovery period, followed by routine cardiovascular care. Immediate postprocedure assessment of hemoglobin and renal function, as well as serial 12-lead electrocardiograms can effectively identify the onset of complications. The documentation of postimplantation echocardiography, completed either at the end of the procedure or before discharge, provides necessary information to determine procedural success and inform long-term follow-up.

Nurse-led accelerated reconditioning

In the absence of postprocedure complications, the focus of care shifts to ensuring patients return to their baseline status as soon as possible and prepare for safe discharge home. With a goal of next-day discharge, every hour counts to accelerate this reconditioning. Nurse-led early mobilization is a central component of postprocedure care. The progressive steps include (1) bedrest flat × 2 hours, (2) bedrest with head of bed elevated to 30° × 2 hours, (3) assistance for first mobilization with progression from sitting at side to walking to toilet after 4 to 6 hours in the absence of complications, and (4) goal of mobilization × 2 on procedure day, including up in chair for evening meal. In addition, rapid resumption of oral fluids and nutrition plays a pivotal role in reducing the risks of deconditioning.[25]

Communication, patient teaching, and discharge

All postprocedure efforts should be focused on maintaining patients on the clinical pathway and addressing potential complications early and effectively. This requires seamless communication between nursing and the implanting team that enables nurses to raise their concerns in a timely way. In-hospital communication with the patient and their family should build on early discharge planning, with confirmation of the individualized planning for safe transition home, and the availability of social support for the first days at home as required. Patient teaching focused on vascular access site care, medications, progressive activity protocol, when to seek help, and follow-up instructions can be provided in a streamlined format using standardized resources. Last, confirmation of readiness for next-day or subsequent discharge can be guided by the following criteria:

1. Absence of persistent (>3 hours) intraventricular conduction delay
2. Absence of diagnostic contraindication (ie, stable hemoglobin and renal function)
3. Return to baseline mobilization
4. Availability of family member for 24 hours to remain with patient

Importantly, patients should hear consistent messages, from every health care provider, at every encounter from referral to discharge to achieve safe and early discharge home. The key messages outlined in **Box 1** must be repeated and endorsed by all providers to clarify expectations and carry individualized discharge planning.

Last, there is growing interest in accelerating physical functioning in the early recovery period. The health benefits of exercise after TAVR are well documented and represent the foundation of cardiac rehabilitation.[39,40] Cardiac rehabilitation in patients after TAVR is safe, reduces mortality, and improves quality of life and exercise tolerance.[41] The 2019 Canadian Cardiovascular Society Position Statement recommends cardiac rehabilitation as a component of long-term management.[42] To date, cardiac rehabilitation has been dramatically underused, and different methods for its delivery (eg, centered-based, home-based, telehealth) have been explored to overcome the presence of barriers to utilization, including referrals and adherence. Regardless of method of delivery, systematic and standardized referrals, combined with patient education regarding the importance of cardiac rehabilitation in the postprocedure recovery, are evidence-based interventions that aim to improve outcomes.

CLINICS CARE POINTS

- Complications after transcatheter aortic valve replacement are increasingly rare; nevertheless, nurses need to be vigilant to identify stroke, hemodynamic instability, acute kidney injury, new conduction delay, and bleeding.

- There is strong evidence that a standardized clinical pathway that prioritizes close monitoring, accelerated nurse-led reconditioning, communication, patient teaching, and criteria-driven discharge is effective to facilitate safe next-day discharge home after transcatheter aortic valve replacement.

SUMMARY

The adoption of best practices along the preprocedure, periprocedure, and post-procedure components of TAVR care is informed by contemporary evidence on how to best care for this patient population. It also reflects the essential need to "get it right, for every patient, at every touch point" to ensure TAVR continues to offer the best possible outcomes, irrespective of individual risk profiles. Nurses are increasingly developing the specialized competencies to support patients' journey of care and to play an essential role to reach these goals and help patients achieve outstanding outcomes. The close scrutiny of the care of TAVR patients offers new opportunities to leverage this evidence across cardiac and other patient populations, and to pursue nurses' collective goal of improving outcomes and efficient health services.

REFERENCES

1. Lauck SB, Wood DA, Baumbusch J, et al. Vancouver transcatheter aortic valve replacement clinical pathway: minimalist approach, standardized care, and discharge criteria to reduce length of stay. Circ Cardiovasc Qual Outcomes 2016;9(3):312–21. Available at. https://www-ncbi-nlm-nih-gov.ezproxy.library.ubc.ca/pubmed/27116975.
2. Kolkailah AA, Doukky R, Pelletier MP, et al. Transcatheter aortic valve implantation versus surgical aortic valve replacement for severe aortic stenosis in people with low surgical risk. Cochrane Libr 2019;2019(12):CD013319. Available at. https://www.cochranelibrary.com/cdsr/doi/10.1002/14651858.CD013319.pub2.
3. Kundi H, Strom JB, Valsdottir LR, et al. Trends in isolated surgical aortic valve replacement according to hospital-based transcatheter aortic valve replacement volumes. JACC Cardiovasc Interv 2018;11(21):2148–56. https://doi.org/10.1016/j.jcin.2018.07.002. Available at.
4. Lauck S, Forman J, Borregaard B, et al. Facilitating transcatheter aortic valve implantation in the era of COVID-19: recommendations for programmes. Eur J Cardiovasc Nurs 2020;19(6):537–44. Available at. https://journals.sagepub.com/doi/full/10.1177/1474515120934057.
5. Santana MJ, Manalili K, Jolley RJ, et al. How to practice person-centred care: a conceptual framework. Health Expect 2018;21(2):429–40. Available at. https://onlinelibrary.wiley.com/doi/abs/10.1111/hex.12640.
6. Hawkey MC, Lauck SB, Perpetua EM, et al. Transcatheter aortic valve replacement program development: recommendations for best practice. Catheter Cardiovasc Interv 2014;84(6):859–67. Available at. https://onlinelibrary.wiley.com/doi/abs/10.1002/ccd.25529.
7. Hawkey M, Højberg Kirk B. The valve program clinician. In: Hawkey M, Lauck S, Perpetua E, et al, editors. Transcatheter aortic valve implantation: a guide for the heart team. Philadelphia PA: Wolters Kluwer; 2020.
8. Perpetua EM, Clarke SE, Guibone KA, et al. Surveying the landscape of structural heart disease coordination: an exploratory study of the coordinator role. Struct

Heart 2019;3(3):201–10. Available at. http://www.tandfonline.com/doi/abs/10.1080/24748706.2019.1581962.

9. Jepma P, Latour CHM, ten Barge, et al. Experiences of frail older cardiac patients with a nurse-coordinated transitional care intervention - a qualitative study. BMC Health Serv Res 2021;21(1):786. Available at. https://www.narcis.nl/publication/RecordID/oai:hbokennisbank.nl:amsterdam_pure:oai:pure.hva.nl:publications%2Ff3e84eac-5ccb-48a3-a246-daf7e735ef4b.

10. Borregaard B, Dahl JS, Lauck SB, et al. Association between frailty and self-reported health following heart valve surgery. Int J Cardiol. Heart & Vasculature 2020;31:100671. https://doi.org/10.1016/j.ijcha.2020.100671. Available at.

11. Frantzen AT, Eide LSP, Fridlund B, et al. Frailty status and patient-reported outcomes in octogenarians following transcatheter or surgical aortic valve replacement. Heart Lung Circ 2021;30(8):1221–31. https://doi.org/10.1016/j.hlc.2020.10.024. Available at.

12. Afilalo J, Lauck S, Kim DH, et al. Frailty in older adults undergoing aortic valve replacement: the FRAILTY-AVR study. J Am Coll Cardiol 2017;70(6):689–700.

13. Forcillo J, Condado JF, Ko Y, et al. Assessment of commonly used frailty markers for high- and extreme-risk patients undergoing transcatheter aortic valve replacement. Ann Thorac Surg 2017;104(6):1939–46. https://doi.org/10.1016/j.athoracsur.2017.05.067. Available at.

14. Lauck SB, Lewis KB, Borregaard B, et al. What is the right decision for me?" integrating patient perspectives through shared decision-making for valvular heart disease therapy. Can J Cardiol 2021;37(7):1054–63.

15. Coylewright M, Palmer R, O'Neill ES, et al. Patient-defined goals for the treatment of severe aortic stenosis: a qualitative analysis. Health Expect 2016;19(5):1036–43.

16. Wood DA, Lauck SB, Cairns JA, et al. The Vancouver 3M (multidisciplinary, multi-modality, but minimalist) clinical pathway facilitates safe next-day discharge home at low-, medium-, and high-volume transfemoral transcatheter aortic valve replacement centers: the 3M TAVR study. JACC Cardiovasc Interv 2019;12(5):459–69. Available at. https://www-ncbi-nlm-nih-gov.ezproxy.library.ubc.ca/pubmed/30846085.

17. Cribier A, Eltchaninoff H, Tron C, et al. Treatment of calcific aortic stenosis with the percutaneous heart valve: mid-term follow-up from the initial feasibility studies: the French experience. J Am Coll Cardiol 2006;47(6):1214–23. Available at. http://content.onlinejacc.org/cgi/content/abstract/47/6/1214.

18. Jensen Hanna A, PhD MD, Condado JF, et al. Minimalist transcatheter aortic valve replacement: the new standard for surgeons and cardiologists using trans-femoral access? J Thorac Cardiovasc Surg 2015;150(4):833–40. Available at. https://www.clinicalkey.es/playcontent/1-s2.0-S0022522315012969.

19. Spaziano M, Lefèvre T, Romano M, et al. Transcatheter aortic valve replacement in the catheterization laboratory versus hybrid operating room: insights from the France TAVI registry. JACC Cardiovasc Interv 2018;11(21):2195–203. Available at. https://www.ncbi.nlm.nih.gov/pubmed/30409276.

20. Lauck S, Wood DA, Sathananthan J, et al. Anesthesia for TAVR patients: should we focus on goals of care? Struct Heart 2020;4(4):310–1. Available at. http://www.tandfonline.com/doi/abs/10.1080/24748706.2020.1774950.

21. Feistritzer H, Kurz T, Stachel G, et al. Impact of anesthesia strategy and valve type on clinical outcomes after transcatheter aortic valve replacement. J Am Coll Cardiol 2021;77(17):2204–15. Available at. https://www.ncbi.nlm.nih.gov/pubmed/33926657.

22. Lauck SB, Kwon J, Wood DA, et al. Avoidance of urinary catheterization to minimize in-hospital complications after transcatheter aortic valve implantation: an observational study. Eur J Cardiovasc Nurs 2018;17(1):66–74. Available at. https://journals.sagepub.com/doi/full/10.1177/1474515117716590.

23. Hinterbuchner L, Coelho S, Esteves R, et al. A cardiac catheterisation laboratory core curriculum for the continuing professional development of nurses and allied health professions (EAPCI) 2016. EuroIntervention 2017;12(16):2028–30. Available at. https://www.ncbi.nlm.nih.gov/pubmed/27821376.

24. Shirey M. Lewin's theory of planned change as a strategic resource. J Nurs Adm 2013;43(2):69–72. Available at. http://ovidsp.ovid.com/ovidweb.cgi?T=JS&NEWS=n&CSC=Y&PAGE=fulltext&D=ovft&AN=00005110-201302000-00005.

25. Lauck SB, Sathananthan J, Park J, et al. Post-procedure protocol to facilitate next-day discharge: results of the multidisciplinary, multimodality but minimalist TAVR study. Catheter Cardiovasc Interv 2020;96(2):450–8. Available at. https://onlinelibrary.wiley.com/doi/abs/10.1002/ccd.28617.

26. Arnold SV, Zhang Y, Baron SJ, et al. Impact of short-term complications on mortality and quality of life after transcatheter aortic valve replacement. JACC: Cardiovascular Interventions 2019;12(4):362–9.

27. Grube E, Sinning J. The "Big Five" complications after transcatheter aortic valve replacement: do we still have to be afraid of them? JACC Cardiovasc Interv 2019; 12(4):370–2. https://doi.org/10.1016/j.jcin.2018.12.019. Available at.

28. Davlouros PA, Mplani VC, Koniari I, et al. Transcatheter aortic valve replacement and stroke: a comprehensive review. J Geriatr Cardiol 2018;15(1):95–104. Available at. https://www.ncbi.nlm.nih.gov/pubmed/29434631.

29. Carroll JD, Mack MJ, Vemulapalli S, et al. STS-ACC TVT registry of transcatheter aortic valve replacement. J Am Coll Cardiol 2020;76(21):2492–516. https://doi.org/10.1016/j.jacc.2020.09.595. Available at.

30. Giustino G, Mehran R, Veltkamp R, et al. Neurological outcomes with embolic protection devices in patients undergoing transcatheter aortic valve replacement: a systematic review and meta-analysis of randomized controlled trials. JACC Cardiovasc Interv 2016;9(20):2124–33. Available at. https://www.ncbi.nlm.nih.gov/pubmed/27765306.

31. Lerakis S, Hayek SS, Douglas PS. Paravalvular aortic leak after transcatheter aortic valve replacement: current knowledge. Circulation 2013;127(3):397–407. Available at. https://www.ncbi.nlm.nih.gov/pubmed/23339094.

32. Peillex M, Marchandot B, Matsushita K, et al. Acute kidney injury and acute kidney recovery following transcatheter aortic valve replacement. PLoS One 2021; 16(8):e0255806. Available at. https://search.proquest.com/docview/2560296229.

33. Adachi Y, Yamamoto M, Shimura T, et al. Late kidney injury after transcatheter aortic valve replacement. Am Heart J 2021;234:122–30. https://doi.org/10.1016/j.ahj.2021.01.007. Available at.

34. Rodés-Cabau J, Muntané-Carol G, Philippon F. Managing conduction disturbances after TAVR: toward a tailored strategy. JACC Cardiovasc Interv. 2021; 14(9):992–4. https://doi.org/10.1016/j.jcin.2021.03.053. Available at.

35. Auffret V, Puri R, Urena M, et al. Conduction disturbances after transcatheter aortic valve replacement: current status and future perspectives. Circulation 2017;136(11):1049–69. Available at. https://www.ncbi.nlm.nih.gov/pubmed/28893961.

36. Scarsini R, De Maria GL, Joseph J, et al. Impact of complications during transfemoral transcatheter aortic valve replacement: how can they be avoided and

managed? J Am Heart Assoc 2019;8(18):e013801. Available at. https://www.ncbi.nlm.nih.gov/pubmed/31522627.

37. Généreux P, Piazza N, Alu MC, et al. Valve academic research consortium 3: updated endpoint definitions for aortic valve clinical research. J Am Coll Cardiol 2021;77(21):2717–46. https://doi.org/10.1016/j.jacc.2021.02.038. Available at.

38. Sathananthan J, Webb JG, Polderman J, et al. Safety of accelerated recovery on a cardiology ward and early discharge following minimalist TAVR in the catheterization laboratory: the Vancouver accelerated recovery clinical pathway. Struct Heart 2019;3(3):229–35. Available at: https://doi.org/10.1080/24748706.2019.1592268. Accessed Oct 21, 2021.

39. Anayo L, Rogers P, Long L, et al. Exercise-based cardiac rehabilitation for patients following open surgical aortic valve replacement and transcatheter aortic valve implant: a systematic review and meta-analysis. Open Heart 2019;6(1):e000922. https://doi.org/10.1136/openhrt-2018-000922. Available at.

40. Pressler A, Förschner L, Hummel J, et al. Long-term effect of exercise training in patients after transcatheter aortic valve implantation: follow-up of the SPORT:TAVI randomised pilot study. Eur J Prev Cardiol 2018;25(8):794–801. Available at. https://journals.sagepub.com/doi/full/10.1177/2047487318765233.

41. Sperlongano S, Renon F, Bigazzi MC, et al. Transcatheter aortic valve implantation: the new challenges of cardiac rehabilitation. J Clin Med 2021;10(4):810. Available at. https://www.ncbi.nlm.nih.gov/pubmed/33671340.

42. Asgar AW, Ouzounian M, Adams C, et al. 2019 Canadian Cardiovascular Society Position statement for transcatheter aortic valve implantation. Can J Cardiol 2019;35(11):1437–48. Available at. https://search.datacite.org/works/10.1016/j.cjca.2019.08.011.

43. Fried LP, Tangen CM, Walston J, et al. Frailty in older adults: evidence for a phenotype. Journals Gerontol Ser A: Biol Sci Med Sci 2001;56(3):M146–57.

44. Guralnik JM, Ferrucci L, Simonsick EM, et al. Lower-extremity function in persons over the age of 70 years as a predictor of subsequent disability. New Engl J Med 1995;332(9):556–62. Available at. http://content.nejm.org/cgi/content/abstract/332/9/556.

45. Rockwood K, Song X, MacKnight C, et al. A global clinical measure of fitness and frailty in elderly people. Can Med Assoc J 2005;173(5):489–95. Available at. http://www.cmaj.ca/cgi/content/abstract/173/5/489.

46. Schoufour JD, Erler NS, Jaspers D-L, et al. Design of a frailty index among community living middle-aged and older people: the rotterdam study. Maturitas 2016;97:14–20. Available at. https://www.clinicalkey.es/playcontent/1-s2.0-S0378512216304145.

Transition to Practice

Implementing Healthy Work Environment Standards through Nurse Resident-Led Evidence-based Practice Change in Transcatheter Aortic Valve Replacement Care on a Cardiac Telemetry Unit

Nicole Judice Jones, MN, APRN, ACNS-BC, CV-BC, CCNS, CHFN, AACC[a],*,
Nina Boutte, RN[b], Kimberly Sanders, RN[b],
Candice Waguespack, BSN, RN, CHFN[b], Stacey Moldthan, RN, CHFN[c],
Patricia O'Leary, BSN, RN-BC[c]

KEYWORDS

- Transition to practice • Nurse residency • Evidence-based practice
- Healthy work environment • Transcatheter aortic valve replacement (TAVR) fast track

KEY POINTS

- The 6 healthy work environment standards are skilled communication, true collaboration, effective decision-making, appropriate staffing, meaningful recognition, and authentic leadership.
- Implementation of healthy work environment standards improves the practice environment for nurses, including new graduate nurses during transition to practice, and can impact nurse satisfaction and retention.
- Evidence-based practice projects are a common component of nurse residency programs, and enhance self-efficacy of new graduate nurses in appraising and integrating evidence into practice.
- Integrating clinical care teams with nurse residents conducting evidence-based practice investigations may facilitate shared decision-making, in addition to the other healthy work environment standards.

[a] East Jefferson General Hospital, Heart Failure and Structural Heart, 4200 Houma Boulevard, Metairie, LA 70006, USA; [b] Cardiac Telemetry Unit, East Jefferson General Hospital, 4200 Houma Boulevard, Metairie, LA 70006, USA; [c] Cardiac Rehab Department, East Jefferson General Hospital, 4200 Houma Boulevard, Metairie, LA 70006, USA
* Corresponding author.
E-mail address: Nicole.jones4@lcmchealth.org

Crit Care Nurs Clin N Am 34 (2022) 233–240
https://doi.org/10.1016/j.cnc.2022.02.012

BACKGROUND OF EVIDENCE-BASED PRACTICE AS AN ESSENTIAL PART OF TRANSITION TO PRACTICE

The transition from nursing school to practice can be a stressful period of adjustment and skill building. When a health care organization's new graduate nurses do not feel supported during this transition to practice, the organization can experience high turnover of these precious nursing resources, and some entry-level nurses leave the profession entirely. Just more than a decade ago, the Future of Nursing publication highlighted the need for nurse residency programs to ameliorate some of the hardships during transition to practice.[1] Nurse residency programs were defined as "planned, comprehensive periods of time during which nursing graduates can acquire the knowledge and skills to deliver safe, quality care." Through the supportive experience of a nurse residency program, however, organizations can decrease turnover of valuable new graduate nurses, improve staffing and efficiency, and promote patient safety. Nurse residencies have been shown to help new graduate nurses to prioritize care, develop critical thinking and decision-making skills, and incorporate research-based evidence into their clinical practice. See **Box 1** for an outline of the strategies detailed in this article.

The American Nurses Credentialing Center promotes nursing excellence and quality outcomes through a Practice Transition Accreditation Program.[2] One method suggested by the American Nurses Credentialing Center to demonstrate professional development that leads to quality outcomes is for nurse residents to conduct evidence-based practice projects. Evidence-based practice projects facilitate the search for and integration of research evidence with clinical expertise to answer a clinical practice question. The Practice Transition Accreditation Program also encourages the facilitation of nurse residents working as part of an interprofessional team to engage in evidence-based practice and quality improvement changes to improve patient outcomes and share the results of these projects.

In a research survey of 127 nursing research leaders in magnet hospitals in the United States in 2020, 1 of the top 3 uses of the evidence-based practice model is through the nurse residency program.[3] The implementation of the findings of an evidence-based practice project is often the responsibility of the primary lead for the project with support from leaders, shared governance councils, mentors, and

---

Box 1
Outline of strategies for successful incorporation of evidence-based practice into a transition to practice program

- Conducting an evidence-based practice project
- Nurse residents work as part of an interprofessional team to implement evidence-based practice
- Nurse residents should share the results of their projects with colleagues
- Support from nurse leaders, educators, shared governance councils, and advanced practice registered nurses are essential
- Nurse resident mentors are critical for vicarious learning, feedback, and encouragement
- The ideal timing of an evidence-based practice project may begin after 6 months of nurse residency
- The delivery of evidence-based practice concepts should be in a structured environment, but individualized to the nurse residents and their nursing specialty and interests

Data from Refs.[2–6]

advanced practice registered nurses. Some of the facilitators of the implementation of evidence-based practice findings are nursing leadership, sharing and disseminating findings, engaged and educated nurses, shared governance, communication and collaboration, mentors, and being a magnet facility. The authors encourage nurse leaders to ensure support for evidence-based practice in all areas where nursing is practiced. Evidence-based practice education and the requirement to complete an evidence-based practice project in nurse residency programs may promote the enculturation of evidence-based practice throughout the organization.

The topic of evidence-based practice projects facilitated by mentors was also highlighted in a review of the literature as a best practice within nurse residency programs.[4] Trained evidence-based practice mentors helped to guide nurse residents through the professional development activity through assistance and feedback during structured sessions. Many research articles reviewed echoed the benefits of evidence-based practice projects in promoting teamwork, autonomous decision-making, and professional development. Nurse leaders, educators, and nurse residency directors are encouraged to focus on quality, safety, and evidence-based practice to aide new graduate nurses in making an effective transition to practice, resulting in improved patient outcomes.

Although many agree on the need for evidence-based practice curricula and projects as part of a new graduate nurse's transition to practice, the ideal timing of such information has been questioned. One correlational study using evidence-based practice learning modules during a 6-month nurse residency program recommended extending nurse residency programs to 1 year to optimize evidence-based practice learning.[5] The study reflects the outcomes of nurse residents at a single organization who were assigned evidence-based practice articles to read and evidence-based practice modules. A positive correlation was found between the nurse residents who read more evidence-based practice articles and higher ratings of critical appraisal of literature, sharing of information with colleagues, and attitudes about changing practice based on evidence. As a whole, the nurse residents experienced improvement in evidence-based practice skills such as forming a research question, retrieving evidence, and disseminating ideas to colleagues, but they were not more likely to do so. The nurse residents' readiness to implement evidence-based practice skills showed great variation. This situation led the author to recommend that evidence-based practice curricula be implemented after the first 6 months of transition to practice as part of a year-long nurse residency program. She also recommended individualization of the education, structured delivery of the information, and the incorporation of specialty knowledge.

A quasiexperimental pretest and post-test study of 66 nurse residents at 2 hospitals revealed improvements in evidence-based practice self-efficacy and likelihood to implement evidence-based practice through use of the Advancing Research through Close Collaboration model.[6] The Advancing Research through Close Collaboration uses evidence-based practice mentors. The author offers evidence-based strategies for integrating evidence-based practice into nurse residency programs to maximize these outcomes. The implementation of an evidence-based practice project during the second one-half of the year-long nurse residency programs increased self-efficacy through mastery experience, vicarious learning with the evidence-based practice mentor from the nurse resident's clinical area, and positive encouragement. A mid-residency survey revealed that the nurse residents' outcome expectancy was lower at the 6-month mark where stress and anxiety about transition to practice have been known to peak. It improved again at the end of the year-long residency, which may support the findings of the correlational study. The author recommends

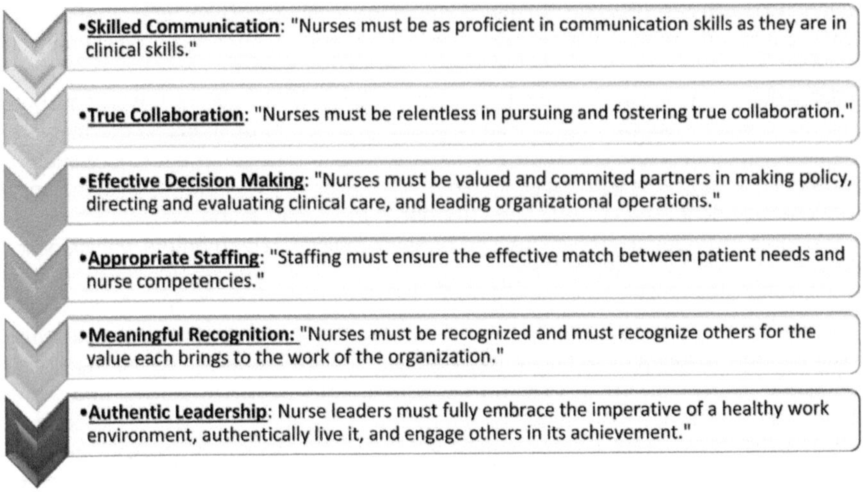

•**Skilled Communication**: "Nurses must be as proficient in communication skills as they are in clinical skills."

•**True Collaboration**: "Nurses must be relentless in pursuing and fostering true collaboration."

•**Effective Decision Making**: "Nurses must be valued and commited partners in making policy, directing and evaluating clinical care, and leading organizational operations."

•**Appropriate Staffing**: "Staffing must ensure the effective match between patient needs and nurse competencies."

•**Meaningful Recognition:** "Nurses must be recognized and must recognize others for the value each brings to the work of the organization."

•**Authentic Leadership**: Nurse leaders must fully embrace the imperative of a healthy work environment, authentically live it, and engage others in its achievement."

Fig. 1. Healthy work environment standards.[7]

evidence-based practice project development over a full year as part of a nurse residency program, which allows for mastery of evidence-based practice skills, mentoring (including sharing of vicarious experiences implementing evidence-based practice), and meaningful recognition and feedback reinforcing new evidence-based practice skills.

HEALTHY WORK ENVIRONMENT

The American Association of Critical Care Nurses published the American Association of Critical Care Nurses Standards for Establishing and Sustaining Healthy Work Environment in 2005 and its second edition in 2016 with the goal of improving patient safety and excellent nursing outcomes.[7] The 6 healthy work environment standards are skilled communication, true collaboration, effective decision-making, appropriate staffing, meaningful recognition, and authentic leadership, and are defined in **Fig. 1**. At a magnet-designated suburban hospital in the Southeastern United States, the healthy work environment standards were used to enhance the transition to practice for nurse residents on a cardiac telemetry unit through an evidence-based practice project aimed at improving the care of patients undergoing transcatheter aortic valve replacement (TAVR).

The nurse residents completed an evidence-based practice project as part of their year-long nurse residency. The residency includes didactic content, discussions, interactive exercises, and emotional support and debriefing. The quality and safety education for nurses competencies are covered, including patient-centered care, teamwork and collaboration, quality improvement, safety, informatics, and evidence-based practice. Although the work of the evidence-based practice project typically occurs during the second half of the residency, concepts about evidence-based practice are introduced throughout the program during structured sessions. The nurse residents were assigned a trained evidence-based practice mentor, who is an advanced practice registered nurse. Nurse residents are expected to disseminate the findings from their evidence-based practice projects and the resulting practice change recommendations during a semiannual evidence-based practice poster showcase.

In an effort to engage nurse residents in their evidence-based practice projects, they are encouraged to develop an evidence-based practice question that arises from their clinical specialty practice or relates to their clinical unit. These nurse residents were interested in implementing a TAVR fast track on the cardiac telemetry unit where they practice. They had access to data from the TAVR quality registry, which showed a hospital length of stay that met the national benchmark for median length of stay, yet all of the TAVR patients were being admitted to critical care. They saw an opportunity to appropriately select patients with specific characteristics that would make them candidates for a TAVR fast track outside of critical care. Their question was, "Would a TAVR fast track checklist identify adult inpatient eligibility for telemetry care versus traditional intensive care, while avoiding an increase in bleeding, vascular complications, and/or mortality?" This evidence-based practice project became much larger than a fast track checklist, because the creation of the checklist required a considerable review of the literature.

TAVR is a procedure offered to patients with severe, symptomatic aortic stenosis as an alternative to an open chest cut and sew valve replacement with a median sternotomy. In TAVR, access is most often gained through the femoral artery in the groin and a new aortic valve is delivered over a catheter that makes its way through the aorta, around the aortic arch, and is deployed inside of the patient's native calcified, stenotic valve. Originally, TAVR was offered to older, more frail patients who were not surgical candidates, but as the technology has progressed and more evidence has been generated, TAVR is now an option for many patients with intermediate-risk and even low-risk status for an open chest aortic valve replacement. Shared decision-making with the patient has become key; the providers on the heart valve team partner with the patient and his loved ones to come to an informed choice of the available and reasonable options.

Some of these lower risk patients may no longer require critical care observation for the first day after TAVR, and some recovery time paired with a stay on the cardiac telemetry unit staffed with highly trained nurses and clinicians is a reasonable alternative. After TAVR, patients are monitored for possible complications from the procedure, including neurologic changes indicating stroke, signs of volume overload and heart failure, cardiac conduction abnormalities, bleeding, and vascular complications. Increasing evidence about optimal care after TAVR allows for clinical pathways that may make care more efficient, less resource intensive, and more comfortable for the patient and family on a cardiac telemetry unit after careful risk stratification.

The nurse residents reviewed and critiqued studies about next day discharge, minimalist TAVR, TAVR fast track, expert consensus decision pathways for TAVR, published clinical pathways for TAVR published by experienced organizations and programs, conduction disturbances after TAVR, delirium after TAVR, potential complications, and recommendations for professional development for nurses and the interprofessional team.

The outcome of the nurse resident-led evidence-based practice project was a TAVR fast track checklist aimed at the risk stratification of appropriate patients to a cardiac telemetry unit instead of critical care, without increasing complications. The nurse residents made recommendations for these education, implementation, and nursing care standards to be incorporated into a clinical pathway. Their recommendations were discussed within the TAVR team, including the heart valve physicians for input and consensus.

SKILLED COMMUNICATION

The nurse residents used communication skills honed during the nurse residency program to communicate the importance of this project. They engaged in respectful communication with the residency coordinators and evidence-based practice team to hear all relevant perspectives while conveying their knowledge and expertise about the care of cardiac patients on their units. The evidence-based practice project team engaged in frequent communication to build consensus and mutual understanding. The nurse residents' ultimate goal of excellent nursing care and safety for patients undergoing TAVR was a focus of all communication and consensus in nursing care.

TRUE COLLABORATION

When true collaboration is used, the unique knowledge and skills of each professional are valued to achieve optimal outcomes for the patient. For each healthy work environment standard, the previous standard(s) are prerequisites, as skilled communication must also be used to achieve true collaboration. The American Association of Critical Care Nurses' critical care nurse work environment surveys show that collaboration with physicians and administrators are key to creating and maintaining a healthy work environment.[7] The nurse residents collaborated with the unit director, who fully supported their efforts and gave them positive feedback throughout the project. The nurse residents also collaborated with the TAVR team physicians, who listened respectfully to their insights, engaged in respectful dialogue, gave them valuable feedback, and ultimately commended them on their work that will lead to improvement in quality patient care. In addition to collaborating with administrators and physicians, the nurse residents collaborated with some of the interprofessional TAVR team members during this project. This situation was unique, because most nurse resident evidence-based practice projects are conducted by groups of nurse residents alone. During this project, other members of the interprofessional team, including an experienced nurse preceptor and mentor from the residents' clinical unit, an advanced practice registered nurse from the TAVR team, and 2 experienced cardiac rehabilitation nurses, attended the nurse residency sessions when the evidence-based practice project was worked on. All team members agreed at the onset of the project that the nurse residents were the leaders of the evidence-based practice project.

EFFECTIVE DECISION-MAKING

Through this evidence-based practice[7] project, the nurse residents lived the healthy work environment standard effective decision-making. The nurse residents were able to find, critique, synthesize, and make decisions about care using the research evidence. As clinical nurses and recent graduates, they were in a prime position to guide decisions about care in collaboration with the interprofessional team and leaders. Their input for the implementation of changes in care will continue to be invaluable as the clinical changes are made. Clinical nurse involvement in decision-making about patient care leads to nurse satisfaction and improved patient outcomes.[7]

APPROPRIATE STAFFING

The appropriate staffing standard states that the needs of the patient are matched by the nurse's competencies. As a part of the implementation plan for the outcome of this evidence-based practice project, nurse education and skill building will be required. The nurse residents who led the evidence-based practice project gave input into the content, methods, and depth of this education as clinical nurses practicing on the cardiac telemetry unit. Through their true collaboration with the unit director and the TAVR team, nurse to patient ratios are also being evaluated to facilitate optimal care using the new TAVR fast track.

MEANINGFUL RECOGNITION

The nurse residents leading this evidence-based practice project have been recognized informally on their clinical unit for their leadership in this project and its resultant improvement in patient care. Near the completion of their evidence-based practice project, they were invited with the project team to attend a TAVR procedure in the control room of the hybrid surgical suite. The TAVR team physicians used skilled communication after the case to discuss their recommendations for care based on the research evidence reviewed, true collaboration to give thoughtful feedback, and meaningful recognition to acknowledge the important work of the nurse residents and their interprofessional evidence-based practice team. As the physicians commended the nurse residents and team and communicated their genuine appreciation, it was clear that the recognition was meaningful to the nurse residents. Additional meaningful recognition was incorporated into the semiannual evidence-based practice poster showcase. The nurse residents' posters are displayed alongside other nursing, allied health, and interprofessional posters and are judged for their scholarship by nurse research leaders, nurse executives, physicians, nursing instructors from collaborating schools of nursing, and the evidence-based practice and research shared governance team. The TAVR fast track poster was selected by the judges as the second place poster, an achievement that is further rewarded with a generous professional development scholarship to be used by the poster authors. One of the nurse residents is enrolled in an RN-to-BSN program, and board certification goals have also been discussed for the timeframe when the nurse residents qualify to sit for examinations.

AUTHENTIC LEADERSHIP

The nurse director for the clinical unit where the nurse residents practice supported them throughout the evidence-based practice project. From encouraging the question development through the project and into the hybrid surgical suite control room, she was a steady source of support and encouragement. She anticipated potential barriers to the successful implementation of the education and new process. She thoughtfully advised the team and physicians of her recommendations for delaying implementation until after the required education and meetings related to a previously planned electronic medical record conversion project to ensure the success of the TAVR care improvement. She continues to express her support and enthusiasm for nursing professional development offerings, as well as advocating for appropriate staffing to support this new care enhancement for TAVR patients.

SUMMARY

New graduate nurses are one of a health care organization's most precious resources. They can be supported during the first year of practice through a nurse residency program. Evidence-based practice should be a critical component of a nurse residency and include didactic content, skill building, mentoring, feedback, and completion of an evidence-based practice project relevant to the nurse resident's specialty practice. This approach ensures the new graduate nurse will take these skills into the remainder of his career to find, appraise, integrate, and evaluate practice improvements based on research evidence. Implementation of these strategies using the healthy work environment standards improves the work environment, patient safety, and outcomes for the nurse residents, the interprofessional team, and patients. Nurse leaders, new graduate mentors, educators, advanced practice registered nurses, and residency directors could consider this approach to potentially enhance nurse satisfaction, retention, and patient outcomes.

ACKNOWLEDGMENTS

The authors acknowledge the following clinicians and leaders for their contributions: the TAVR Team physicians: Pedro Cox-Alomar, MPH, MD, FACC, FSCAI; Tod Engelhardt, MD, FACS; and James Perrien, MD; for their true collaboration on this project; nurse residency coordinators: Layne Mistretta, MSN, RN; and Megan Kruse, BSN, RN, CCRN; for facilitating effective decision-making by allowing the clinician team to collaborate during the nurse residency evidence-based practice project breakout sessions; and 2 east/cardiac telemetry unit director: Victoria Johnson, MSN, RN, PCCN, for her authentic leadership in supporting this project and advancing nursing practice on the cardiac telemetry unit.

CLINICS CARE POINTS

- Using the healthy work environment standards as a framework can enhance support for nurse residents.
- Completion of EBP projects facilitates professional development and application of evidence to practice. Optimal timing for these projects is greater than 6 months after starting the nurse residency.
- Didactic content about EBP, skill building, mentor, and feedback should be incorporated.

DISCLOSURE

The authors have nothing to disclose.

REFERENCES

1. Institute of Medicine. The Future of nursing: leading change, advancing health. Washington, DC: The National Academies Press; 2011. https://doi.org/10.17226/12956. Available at.
2. American Nurses Credentialing Center 2021. Practice transition accreditation program application manual. Available at. https://www.nursingworld.org/organizational-programs/accreditation/ptap/download-ptap-manual/. Accessed online October 8, 2021.
3. Speroni K, McLaughlin M, Friesen M. Use of evidence-based practice models and research findings in Magnet-designated hospitals across the United States: national survey results. Worldviews Evidence-Based Nurs 2020;17(2):98–107.
4. Cochran C. Effectiveness and best practice of nurse residency programs: a literature review. MedSurg Nurs 2017;26(1):53–8.
5. Jackson N. Incorporating evidence-based practice learning into a nurse residency program: are new graduates ready to apply evidence at the bedside? J Nurs Adm 2016;46(5):278–83.
6. Smith A. Evidence-based practice training in nurse residency programs: enhancing confidence for practice implementation. Teach Learn Nurs 2021;16:315–20.
7. American Association of Critical Care Nurses. AACN standards for establishing and sustaining healthy work environments: a journey to excellence. 2nd Edition. 2016. Available at. https://www.aacn.org/nursing-excellence/standards/aacn-standards-for-establishing-and-sustaining-healthy-work-environments. [Accessed 8 October 2021]. Accessed online.

Moving?

Make sure your subscription moves with you!

To notify us of your new address, find your **Clinics Account Number** (located on your mailing label above your name), and contact customer service at:

Email: journalscustomerservice-usa@elsevier.com

800-654-2452 (subscribers in the U.S. & Canada)
314-447-8871 (subscribers outside of the U.S. & Canada)

Fax number: 314-447-8029

Elsevier Health Sciences Division
Subscription Customer Service
3251 Riverport Lane
Maryland Heights, MO 63043

*To ensure uninterrupted delivery of your subscription, please notify us at least 4 weeks in advance of move.

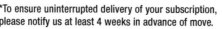